Allergies at your fingertips

THE COMPREHENSIVE ALLERGY REFERENCE BOOK FOR THE YEAR 2000

Dr Joanne Clough DM, FRCA, MRCP, FRCPCH
Senior Lecturer in Paediatric Respiratory Medicine, University of Southampton, and Consultant Paediatrician, Southampton General Hospital

CLASS PUBLISHING · LONDON

Joanne Clough asserts her right as set out in sections 77 and 78 of the Copyright, Designs and Patents Act 1988 to be identified as the author of this work wherever it is published commercially and whenever any adaptation of this work is published or produced, including any sound recordings or films made of or based upon this work.

Printing history
First published 1997
Reprinted with amendments, 1998

The author and the publishers welcome feedback from the users of this book. Please contact the publishers.
Class Publishing (London) Ltd, Barb House, Barb Mews, London W6 7PA
Telephone: 0171 371 2119
Fax: 0171 371 2878 [International +44171]
email: post@class.co.uk
website: http://www.class.co.uk

A CIP record for this book is available from the British Library

ISBN 1 872362 52 4

Designed by Wendy Bann

Edited by Susan Bosanko

Indexed by Valerie Elliston

Cartoons by Jane Taylor

Line illustrations by David Woodroffe

Produced by Landmark Production Consultants Ltd, Princes Risborough

Typesetting by Sally Brock, High Wycombe, Buckinghamshire

Printed and bound in Great Britain by Clays Ltd, St Ives plc

Contents

Acknowledgements   viii
Foreword by Professor Stephen T. Holgate   ix

INTRODUCTION   1
How to use this book   2

CHAPTER 1 *What is allergy?*
Introduction   3
Allergy explained   4
Symptoms   13
Triggers   16
Inheritance   19
The scale of the problem   22

CHAPTER 2 *Asthma*
Introduction   24
Asthma explained   25
Symptoms   30
Triggers   32
Diagnosis and assessment   37
Treatment   42
Asthma and allergy   55

CHAPTER 3 *Skin allergies*
Introduction   61
Skin allergies explained   62
Causes of eczema   69
Treatment for eczema   72
Diet and eczema   80
Living with eczema   83
Dermatitis   87

CHAPTER 4 *Hayfever*
Introduction   93
Hayfever explained   94
Is it really hayfever?   95
Symptoms   97
Triggers   103
Treatment   106
Living with hayfever   115

CHAPTER 5 *Food allergies*
Introduction   120
Food allergy explained   121
Symptoms   130
Triggers   132
Diagnosis   137
Living with food allergies   142
Coeliac disease   148

CHAPTER 6 *Anaphylaxis*
Introduction   151
Anaphylaxis explained   152
Emergency treatment   157
Identifying the cause   162
Living with anaphylaxis   166

CHAPTER 7 *Allergies at work*
Introduction 172
General questions 173
Factory work 175
Working outdoors 180
Office work 182
Other occupations 183

CHAPTER 8 *Living with allergies*
Introduction 188
Holidays and travel 189
School 196
Going into hospital 205
Sex and pregnancy 208
Finance 212
Miscellaneous 213

CHAPTER 9 *Allergen avoidance and complementary therapies*
Introduction 217
Allergen avoidance in general 218
House dust mite 221
Pollens 228
Pet allergens 232
Food allergens 235
Complementary therapies 239

GLOSSARY 247

APPENDIX 1
Diagnosing your allergies 257

APPENDIX 2
Useful addresses 272

APPENDIX 3
Useful publications 276

INDEX 279

Acknowledgements

I am grateful to everyone who has helped in the production of this book, but in particular would like to thank the following:

Lucy Edwards for her invaluable support in the preparation of this manuscript;

Peter Howarth, Mark Levy, Greta Barnes and Sue Ollier for reviewing the manuscript;

Peter Thomas for his contribution, particularly to the chapter on hayfever;

Jane Taylor for drawing such delightful cartoons;

the National Asthma and Respiratory Training Centre for providing the line illustrations of devices that appear in Chapter 2;

members of the British Allergy Foundation for passing on to me questions and queries on allergic problems;

and finally my patients and friends who have allergic disorders for providing me with many of the questions and most of the answers.

Foreword

by Professor Stephen T. Holgate MD, DSc, FRCP

MRC Clinical Professor of Immunopharmacology, University of Southampton

The word 'allergy' was first used in 1906 by Pirquet, who used it to describe an immunological reaction against substances in our environment. This description, however, would be better applied to the whole subject of immunology, and nowadays the term 'allergy' is used specifically to indicate harmful reactions to substances in our everyday environment which produce their effect through mechanisms involving our immune response leading to various types of either acute or chronic inflammation. This description of allergy separates it quite clearly from the many other forms of intolerance that occur to environmental substances, such as reactions to food causing migraine and even 'allergy to the 20th century'.

One of the common features of allergic disorders is that they tend to cluster in families and in any one person may manifest at a number of sites. For example, it is quite common for patients to have asthma, hayfever and eczema together. Thus allergy tends not to affect just a single organ, but multiple organs producing a range of symptoms. It is because of this that allergy fits uncomfortably into the more traditional practice of medicine which involves specialists in particular systems or organs.

This book is a refreshing distillation of the medical literature, written in a question and answer format and designed to help steer patients accurately through the allergy maze. Dr Clough is a child health specialist who has a special interest in asthma, eczema and hayfever, and she therefore is particularly well qualified to translate medical knowledge into a form that is easily understandable by the public.

The rising trends that appear to be occurring in disorders such as asthma and hayfever are almost entirely related to the increasing trends in allergy produced probably by changes in our environment. The importance of environment in helping allergic disorder cannot be underestimated. This book presents a balanced view of how medical intervention coupled with environmental control can lead to improvement in the manifestations of many allergic disorders.

The very practical and sensible approach that Dr Clough has taken in this book will, I am sure, be of tremendous help to those who experience allergic disorders themselves or who have a child with allergies. While the book is not intended as a substitute for consultation with general practitioners or a hospital-based specialist, it certainly does produce excellent first hand guidance as to what to do when confronted by the myriad of questions linked to the symptoms of allergic disorders, especially those which relate to life quality and day-to-day living.

Stephen T. Holgate

Introduction

Allergy is extremely common, with allergies in one form or another affecting one-third of our population. As many as half of all sufferers are children. Despite these problems being so common, misunderstandings about allergy are frequent and misinformation is rife. The enormous number of different ways in which allergic disorders can present themselves may be partly responsible for this confusion: an allergy may occur as an isolated problem such as penicillin allergy; it may be a part of one of the common disorders of the Western world such as asthma, hayfever and eczema; or it may cause a less common illness such as coeliac disease. Some sufferers may be allergic to only one substance, others to a wide variety. The problems caused by allergy may be trivial (such as nettle rash) or they may be life-threatening (such as anaphylaxis), yet it is the same underlying biological mechanism which is responsible for each of these many different conditions.

Although much about allergy is still unknown, we do have a great deal of information which anyone with an allergy-related problem will find useful in the understanding and management of their disorder. With the help of this information, you and your doctor will be able to tackle your allergic problem more effectively. Family and friends may also benefit from learning more about both the causes and the management of allergic problems, as they may then feel more able to offer help and to co-operate with any necessary changes in lifestyle. Accurate interpretation of what is and is not allergy is important: you may realise from reading this book that your problem is not due to allergy, in which case you will then be free to discover the real cause.

I hope that this book will help you to understand the way in which allergies happen, what the common causes of allergies are, and how to manage them effectively, as well as dispelling some of the myths which are so widespread in these areas. If you are well informed and well prepared, I believe you will feel more in control, your allergies will become more manageable, and your enjoyment of life will increase.

How to use this book

Because individual people have very different allergic problems, this book has been designed in a way which means you do not have to read it from cover to cover unless you wish to do so. Instead it can be used selectively to meet your own particular situation. It has a detailed list of contents and a comprehensive index so that you can quickly identify the parts which are relevant to you. Cross references in the text will lead you to more detailed information when this might be useful, and essential information is repeated whenever it seems to be necessary.

Please remember that a book like this cannot provide exact and full answers to your individual problems. What it can do is to provide you with the information which will help you to obtain those answers from doctors and other health professionals.

Not everyone will agree with all the answers I have given, but future editions of this book can only be improved if you let me know where you disagree, or have found the advice to be unhelpful, or if you have any questions which you think I have not covered. Please write to me c/o Class Publishing, Barb House, Barb Mews, London W6 7PA, UK.

1
What is allergy?

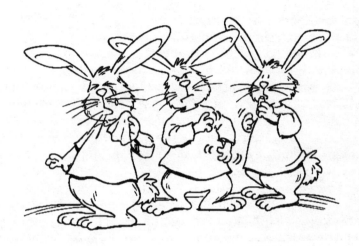

Introduction

Allergy seems to be becoming more common, and the number of people affected is rising every year. The reason for this is not yet clear, but I shall explore some of the possibilities in this chapter. First of all, I want to explain what happens in the body when an allergy occurs, and how to decide whether or not an allergy is the cause of your particular problem. Other sections discuss some of the common substances which can set off the train of events leading to allergy, and answer the questions that are frequently asked about how allergy is inherited.

Allergy explained

Allergy is a term which seems to be used to describe almost any kind of illness these days. What exactly is allergy?

If you have an allergy, it means that your immune system (your body's defence network against outside 'attackers' such as viruses and bacteria) reacts abnormally or inappropriately to a substance which should be harmless.

The term allergy is often used rather loosely to describe any reaction of the body which involves a food or a drug, but many of these reactions (eg nausea after taking certain antibiotics, or diarrhoea in toddlers when they eat certain foods) are due to a predictable side effect and are not allergic in origin. True allergic reactions tend to occur in people who are prone to allergic disorders, a tendency which is described as atopy.

What exactly is atopy?

Atopy is not an illness. It is an inherited feature of someone's constitution which makes that person more likely to develop an allergic disorder. Not everyone who is atopic actually has one of the allergic disorders – which include asthma, eczema, hayfever and perennial allergic rhinitis (a problem similar to hayfever but which lasts all year round) – but all atopic people have inherited the tendency or predisposition to develop them, and might do so in the future.

The reason why atopic people have a tendency to develop allergic disorders is because they have the ability to produce the allergy antibody (called immunoglobulin E or IgE, and discussed in more detail in the answer to the next question) when they come into contact with common substances which would not normally be harmful. The word atopy is a good way of describing this inappropriate reaction, as it is derived from the Greek word 'atopos', which means 'out of place'.

Atopy is a characteristic which tends to run in families and a number of scientists are currently trying to identify the gene on our chromosomes which causes it (genes determine the characteristics which we inherit from our parents, and chromosomes are the structures in our body cells that carry the genes). Identifying the gene would make it easier to carry out research into why allergies happen, how they are inherited, and what we can do to prevent them. In the meantime, your doctor makes the diagnosis of atopy mainly by paying attention to the symptoms you describe, perhaps with the help of some of the tests described in Appendix 1.

Most people in my family are allergic to one thing or another. How do you become allergic to something?

To explain this, I need to start by describing how the immune system works. The immune system is the network within the body that protects us from outside 'attackers', which include viruses, bacteria and parasites, and some forms of injury. This system is usually very efficient at telling the difference between these harmful micro-organisms and other harmless substances which do not pose a threat to your body. When your immune system defends your body against a potentially harmful attacker, it develops a memory of the micro-organism, so that it can be recognised should it attack you again. This memory is in the form of many small structures called antibodies, which are tailor-made for each attacker. Each set of antibodies is unique, and you have a different set of antibodies for every attacker.

There are five different types or classes of antibody. Each type, termed an immunoglobulin, has a different function.

- Immunoglobulin A (abbreviation IgA) is found in secretions such as tears and saliva, and defends us against micro-organisms which might invade our respiratory and digestive systems.
- Immunoglobulin M (IgM) is a temporary type of antibody formed when a new attacker invades your body.
- Immunoglobulin G (IgG) is the antibody which takes over

from IgM to form a lasting (usually lifelong) memory of the attacker.
- Immunoglobulin D (IgD) is a mystery – we know it is there, but we do not know what it does.
- Immunoglobulin E (IgE) is the allergy antibody. People who do not have allergies normally have only small amounts of IgE, but can produce more as a response to parasites such as worms. People with allergies readily produce large amounts of IgE.

If your immune system is working effectively, it is constantly at the ready to eliminate an attacker which it has met before. The tailor-made IgG antibody which has already been made attaches immediately to the attacker, allowing the many other components of the immune system, led by the white blood cells, to destroy it before it can cause an infection. This is why we only suffer once from childhood infections such as chickenpox.

If you are atopic (as discussed in the answer to the previous question), your immune system works perfectly well against these infectious organisms. However, it also has a tendency to react to substances which should be harmless and treat them as if they were attackers. These substances, known as allergens, are mistakenly seen by your immune system as being dangerous, and antibodies of the type known as immunoglobulin E (IgE) are made against them. Once your body has met an allergen, large amounts of IgE are quickly made when it meets the same allergen again, even in the tiniest amounts. This IgE then starts off the series of events which lead to an allergic reaction. This process involves many other components of the immune system, particularly the white blood cells, all of which are co-ordinated by the body's chemical messengers. The end result of this complex chain of events is that the affected parts of the body become inflamed and display the typical symptoms of an allergy – swelling, redness, tenderness or itching, and increased watery secretions.

An allergy cannot happen the first time you come into contact with an allergen. You may even tolerate a substance quite happily for a long time and then, for no apparent reason, develop an allergic reaction to it. Once this has happened, an allergic response will take place each time your body meets that allergen. Your reaction will not necessarily be identical on each occasion: there are many factors which may alter its severity, and the allergy may grow weaker – or indeed stronger – with time. You can see that allergies are not very predictable!

I know that allergies are often treated with antihistamine medicines, but what is histamine?

Histamine is just one (but probably the best known) of the chemicals produced by your body in the course of an allergic reaction, and it causes the symptoms of itching, swelling, redness and mucus production. It is produced by your body as the end result of a large number of messages which are passed in chemical form from one cell to another, a process which begins when your body is in contact with an allergen.

As you say, one of the treatments for allergies is to give drugs which block the action of histamine, called antihistamines. Whilst these drugs are useful, they only suppress the effects of histamine after it has been produced. Treatments which interrupt the allergy process earlier on in its progress are usually more effective (eg the inhaled steroids used in asthma).

My doctor has told me that my bowel problems are caused by a food intolerance, but I'm sure it's all due to an allergy. My husband thinks I've just got a rather sensitive stomach. Are we all just using different words to describe the same thing, or is there really a difference between allergy, intolerance and sensitivity? And does it matter?

Although the term allergy is commonly used to describe any unpleasant reaction to a drug, food, insect sting or chemical, it is more correct to reserve it for the description of a very particular type of reaction, and to use the terms intolerance and sensitivity as follows.

• An intolerance is said to occur when you develop unpleasant symptoms after eating a substance which your body cannot handle adequately. For example, some people have unpleasant symptoms after drinking milk or eating products made from milk. They cannot digest milk and milk products properly because their digestive systems do not produce enough of a particular chemical (an enzyme called lactase) which is needed to break down and digest the sugar in the milk (which is called lactose). The symptoms include crampy abdominal pain and diarrhoea, both of which are due to the presence of undigested milk sugar in the bowel. These symptoms are not allergic in nature, and will not occur if only tiny quantities of milk are drunk. This form of food intolerance is called lactose intolerance, and the answer to it is to avoid milk and milk products.

• A sensitivity is a reaction to a substance which is an exaggeration of a normal side effect produced by that substance. For example, consider salbutamol (brand names Ventolin and Aerolin) which is used in reliever inhalers for asthma. If it is given in a high enough dose, most people will develop shakiness and feel 'revved up'. Some individuals, particularly children, develop these side effects on quite small doses, and can be said to be unusually sensitive to salbutamol (but they are not allergic to it).

• A true allergy is a reaction produced when your body meets a normally harmless substance which has been remembered from a previous exposure, and this reaction involves IgE antibodies (these were discussed in an earlier answer in this section). Once an allergy has developed, even a tiny amount of the allergen can lead to a reaction.

The difference between intolerance, sensitivity and allergy can matter, because if your problem is not correctly diagnosed you may not get the most appropriate and effective treatment for it – for example, antihistamine medications will not help in lactose intolerance. However, if you find that the only suitable treatment for your symptoms is to avoid the substance which is affecting you, then it probably doesn't matter which term you choose to use. In your particular case, it sounds as if you know that there are particular foods which upset you, and you may want to avoid them when you are eating out at a restaurant or a friend's house.

If calling your problem an allergy makes it easier for you to do this, then go ahead!

You will find more information about food allergies in Chapter 5, and about allergen avoidance in Chapter 9.

I have hayfever which affects my nose, my eyes and my chest. I have a friend who has an allergy which affects her skin. Are there any other parts of the body which can be affected by allergies?

Allergic reactions can occur as a generalised reaction involving the skin (urticaria, angioedema) or the whole body (anaphylaxis), or they may be confined to specific parts of the body such as the eyes (allergic conjunctivitis, hayfever), the nose (perennial allergic rhinitis, hayfever), the lungs (asthma), the skin (eczema, contact dermatitis) or the bowel (food allergies). The symptoms of the allergic reaction will vary depending upon which part of the body is affected, but the underlying mechanism of what is happening in the immune system is the same for all of them.

You will find more information on all the allergies mentioned here in other chapters of this book.

I have heard of people suffering from something called total allergy syndrome. What is this, how common is it, and how is it treated?

A number of different terms – including total allergy syndrome and multiple chemical sensitivity – are used to describe a condition in which the sufferer appears to experience reactions to a wide range of substances. The symptoms include memory loss, fatigue, depression, nausea and breathing difficulties. As the substances thought to be responsible include many chemicals, plastics and other synthetics, this is sometimes regarded as an allergy to modern living. Sufferers often find some relief from their symptoms by avoiding exposure to all fumes and chemicals, but this often means that they end up cutting themselves off from everyday life.

Most doctors are reluctant to believe that this condition is in fact due to allergy, and certainly the classic immune response with the production of IgE (discussed earlier in this section) is not involved. However, this does not mean to say that the symptoms are not real, just that they are not caused by allergy. The Department of Health has organised an investigation into the cause of this problem. When the results are available, they may help us to understand the condition.

If my allergies are not treated, will they become worse?

Allergies can vary in their severity over relatively short periods of time, and many allergies become less severe as you grow older. Despite this, if a safe and well-tolerated treatment if available for your allergy then it is better to treat it so that the inflammation in your body's tissues is controlled, and any scarring or other long-term consequences are kept to a minimum.

In a small number of people with allergies an allergy may increase in severity as time goes on, with repeated exposure to the allergen causing more marked symptoms each time. If you are one of these people then it is particularly important for you to avoid the allergen as much as you can, and to take any medications given to you exactly as prescribed by your doctor.

I am allergic to grass pollen. Will I always have this allergy?

Unfortunately the tendency to develop allergy (called atopy, and explained earlier in this section) is written as a permanent message on your chromosomes (the genetic material which you inherit from your parents) and will never go away. However, the likelihood of developing new allergies decreases with age, and often existing allergics become less troublesome as you grow older – elderly people seem to suffer fewer allergic problems. I don't know how old you are, but the good news is that as you get older, your allergy is likely to become less of a problem.

As you know what is responsible for your allergy, you may be able to control your symptoms by minimising your contact with grass pollen (ways of doing this are discussed in the section on *Pollens* in Chapter 9). Alternatively, your symptoms might be reduced to relatively trouble-free levels by a careful choice from the wide range of treatments available, which you should discuss with your doctor. So although you will probably always have the tendency to allergy, there is a chance that you need not always suffer the symptoms.

Can allergies be cured?

No. Most treatments for allergy aim to suppress the symptoms, but none of them is a cure. There is one treatment, called desensitization or allergen immunotherapy, which attempts to eliminate an allergy by making the body more tolerant of the allergen, but this is not a procedure which should be undertaken lightly (nor should it be regarded as a cure for allergy). There are serious risks associated with it, and it needs to be repeated on a long-term basis.

Research is going on at the moment into a vaccine against allergy which might be used to protect children from developing allergies. If the results of this research are successful, the vaccine (made from a micro-organism related to the tuberculosis organism) could be given to babies before they had the chance to become allergic to anything. Unfortunately, such a vaccine is still a long way off and we have as yet no proof that it will work.

What is immunotherapy?

Immunotherapy (desensitization) is a treatment which aims to reduce or even eliminate symptoms of specific allergies by building up the body's tolerance to the allergen responsible for the problem. This is done by giving repeated injections of increasing amounts of the allergen, starting with minute doses. It is only effective against certain types of allergy such as hayfever, certain other seasonal allergies, and anaphylaxis caused by insect stings such as wasp and bee stings. It cannot be used against food and drug allergies, although it is sometimes used to provide temporary protection in rare cases of drug allergy where the drug in question is the only possible form of treatment for a serious illness. It is never appropriate for non-seasonal asthma or perennial allergic rhinitis, or for allergies of the digestive system or skin.

Immunotherapy may take years to achieve results. This means it may need to be a lifelong therapy, and it therefore requires a major commitment. Treatment begins with the injection into the deeper layers of the skin of a very small quantity of the substance to which you are allergic. Each time the injection is repeated, the quantity of the allergen is increased (providing that the previous injection did not produce undue symptoms), until a maintenance level is reached which, without producing problems itself, controls the symptoms of the allergy being treated. Injections are given once or twice a week at first, reducing to once a month after a few months. This treatment must only be given in a hospital by a fully trained doctor, and on each occasion the person receiving treatment must be closely observed for a minimum of two hours, as rarely (about one in every 200 treatments) severe reactions may occur. Women are more likely than men to suffer reactions to this form of treatment, and reactions are more likely if the person is being treated for bee-sting allergy.

My daughter has always had very severe eczema. My doctor now tells me that she has something called hyper-IgE syndrome and has prescribed a drug that my husband takes for his ulcers! Can you explain this to me?

Hyper-immunoglobulin E syndrome (usually abbreviated to hyper-IgE) is a rare condition in which enormous amounts of the immunoglobulin E antibody are produced. This leads to an exaggerated tendency towards allergic disorders, particularly eczema and asthma. We know that histamine, a chemical produced by the body, plays a major role in this problem. That is why the treatment consists of blocking the effects of histamine with antihistamine medicines.

It is not enough just to use the conventional antihistamine medications generally used in hayfever, as these only block some of the actions of histamine (they are known as H_1 blockers). Luckily, a second type of medication has been developed which blocks the other actions of histamine. These H_2 blockers are commonly used for stomach and duodenal (peptic) ulcers. Treatment for hyper-IgE consists of a combination of these two types of antihistamines: a conventional antihistamine such as ketotifen or cetirizine (both H_1 blockers), plus an ulcer drug such as cimetidine or ranitidine (both H_2 blockers). Do persevere with these medications, as it can take up to a year to see the full benefit, although you should begin to see some improvement within a few weeks.

Symptoms

What are the symptoms of allergy, and how do they occur?

There is no such thing as a typical allergic reaction, as the symptoms of allergy can vary enormously between individuals. The response to an allergen might even be different in the same person on two different occasions. To a certain extent, the symptoms you have will depend on which allergen is involved and which parts of your body are affected. A few examples are given here, but this list is not exhaustive.

- If grass pollen is the allergen, then it is your eyes and nose which will be affected. The pollen grains are relatively large and tend to settle on the surface of your eyes and the lining of your nose – which then become red and swollen, and produce an increased amount of secretions (ie you develop a runny nose and weepy eyes).
- A number of allergens – including those from house dust mites, cats and dogs – are very light, and so instead of settling in your nose, they are inhaled down into your lungs, causing a narrowing of your airways. This leads to greater difficulty in moving air in and out of your airways, excess mucus or phlegm production (which blocks your airways even more), and increased irritability in your lungs causing coughing and wheezing.
- If your digestive system is affected by a food allergen, your bowel becomes inflamed and you will experience an increased volume of watery motions (diarrhoea) with spasm or colic of the bowel and sometimes vomiting.

Although these symptoms all seem quite different, they are all caused by the same process of tissue inflammation. Inflammation is your body's natural response to what it perceives as an 'attacker', and the process is designed to protect your body against the spread of an injury or infection. If you are atopic then your body may treat an allergen as an attacker and set up the inflammatory process. To start with, the allergen must gain access to your body, and this is usually through your nose, lungs, skin or bowel. Once there, the IgE (which was made the first time the allergen was encountered) allows the allergen to attach itself to a number of different cells of the immune system. Some of these cells produce chemical messengers which alert other cells in the immune system that an 'attack' is happening and encourage them to gather. Another group of cells produce chemicals which are directly responsible for causing tissue damage resulting in swelling, redness, soreness and itching. Other cells are encouraged to produce more IgE antibodies which will, in their turn, be able to continue the inflammatory process. Without treatment the inflammation may continue indefinitely, even after the allergen has been removed.

You will find more information about atopy and IgE antibodies in the section called *Allergy explained* at the beginning of this chapter.

How do I know if I am allergic to a particular allergen?

If you suspect that you might be allergic to something it is likely that you have experienced a number of symptoms which involve irritation or inflammation of a certain part of your body. To know whether or not an allergy actually is responsible, you should involve your doctor, who will need to consider:

- when your symptoms started;
- whether they occur at particular times of the day or of the year;
- how often they occur;
- which part of your body is affected;
- the type of symptoms you have and how severe they are;
- whether anyone else in your family has allergy-related problems;

- whether or not you have found anything which helps to relieve your symptoms; and
- whether or not there is anything in particular which makes them worse.

Your doctor will then want to examine you. At this stage it might be clear whether your problem is due to an allergy and, if so, which one. If not, you may be referred for further tests (a number of different tests are used to look for evidence of particular allergies, and they are described in Appendix 1).

As the end result of an allergic reaction is inflammation of the affected part of the body, the symptoms of allergy usually involve swelling, soreness, itchiness and increased secretions. Although allergic problems can make you feel tired, irritable and moody, this will always be as a result of the problems caused by inflammation rather than as a symptom on its own (for example, if your asthma is worse, you are likely to sleep less well and then to feel tired and irritable as a consequence). Generalised feelings of tiredness in the absence of specific allergic symptoms are unlikely to be due to allergy.

One indication that an allergy is responsible for your symptoms comes from seeing them improve when the allergen is removed from your environment. However, this cannot always be regarded as an ultimate proof of allergy, for two reasons. The first is that your symptoms might be due to intolerance or sensitivity rather than allergy (the differences between these terms were explained in the previous section in this chapter): avoiding the problem substance would still relieve your symptoms. The second is that is not always possible completely to avoid certain allergens, especially grass pollen and the house dust mite. Should you prove to be allergic to an allergen which cannot be avoided, your doctor will be able offer you one or more of the different medications currently available for the treatment of allergies.

My daughter is unwell whenever she drinks a lot of milk, which makes me think she may be allergic to it. However, my GP says it might not be that, but that instead she may just not be able to tolerate milk. He wants to perform some skin prick tests, but as she is terrified of needles we are

not very keen for her to have to go through that. Why can't our doctor simply tell what is wrong from her symptoms?

Most of the symptoms which our bodies produce as a way of telling us that something is wrong are not specific, that is the same symptoms may be produced by a wide range of different problems or diseases. Because of this, your doctor cannot tell what is wrong with your daughter just from her symptoms. It sounds as if milk is certainly the cause, but whether her problem is an intolerance or an allergy will be difficult to tell without some form of testing. The difference between intolerance and true allergy was discussed in the previous section on *Allergy explained*.

The symptoms of milk intolerance (diarrhoea and abdominal discomfort) tend only to occur if relatively large amounts of milk are taken (small amounts are usually no problem) and the condition is often temporary. If a true allergy to milk is the problem (this usually occurs in younger children), the symptoms will occur even if only a tiny amount of milk is taken. However, the symptoms can be the same as those of milk intolerance.

Although my advice to you would be the same whichever the problem was – to avoid milk in your daughter's diet – I think that it is important to find out whether or not she has an allergy. If she does, you will need to be very strict with her diet and avoid milk completely, something which it is not easy to do (just what is involved is discussed in the section on *Food allergens* in Chapter 9). If she has a milk intolerance, she will be able to take small quantities of milk. Skin prick testing (discussed further in Appendix 1) does not have to involve the use of needles, as small lancets only 1 mm long are usually used, and it does not hurt. I would strongly advise that you allow your doctor to arrange these tests for your daughter.

Triggers

What is an allergen? How many different allergens are there?

An allergen is any substance which acts as a trigger for allergy,

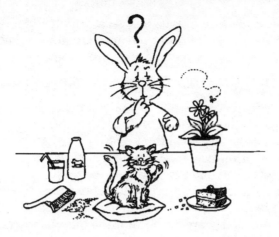

provoking an allergic reaction in someone who is atopic (allergic reactions and atopy are discussed in more detail in the section called *Allergy explained* at the beginning of this chapter). It is impossible to say how many different allergens exist, as almost anything can be an allergen for someone: while I have been writing this book I have been told about allergies to substances as wide-ranging as castor oil plants and ladybird bites.

However, the most common allergens are house dust mites, pollen from trees and grasses, peanut and egg proteins, dog dander (the scales from their hair or fur, something like dandruff in humans), and cat dander (a combination of saliva, which cats use for grooming, and their 'dandruff'). What these all have in common is that they contain protein: for example, the house dust mite allergen is a protein in the mite faeces; pollen is a protein; and there is a protein in cat saliva. Only the protein fragments of food can cause allergies – if peanut oil could be obtained 100% pure (containing only the oil and no protein fragments) then it could not cause peanut allergy. Although we tend to think of protein as part of the food we eat, a protein is in fact an organic compound containing hydrogen, oxygen and nitrogen which forms an important part of all living organisms. There are many, many different proteins, and their importance to life is shown in the name: the word 'protein' comes from the Greek word 'proteios' which means 'primary'.

There are some non-protein allergens, which include penicillin and some other drugs. In order to cause an allergy, these have to be bound to a protein once they are in the body.

Why am I allergic to some things and not to others?

Being atopic does not mean that you will become allergic to any allergen in particular, just that you may, at some stage of your life, develop an allergy to something (atopy is discussed in more detail in the section called *Allergy explained* at the beginning of this chapter). It seems that the way in which you first encounter an allergen is important in determining whether or not you will be allergic to it, as is the scale of your exposure to it, and whether or not you were made more vulnerable at the time by also being exposed to other factors such as tobacco smoke or a respiratory infection. As there are still many aspects of allergy that remain a mystery, we have no way of predicting whether or not you will develop any further allergies.

I have seen a number of advertisements for anti-house dust mite sprays. What is the house dust mite? Does it cause allergies?

The house dust mite is a species of small mite, too small to be seen with the naked eye, which lives on the scales of dead human skin which we all shed all the time. Its Latin name is *Dermatophagoides pteronyssinus*, and it is the commonest type of mite living in house dust, although up to 12 different mite species can be found if the dust is analysed carefully. House dust mites are found in almost all homes in this country, because they love the relatively warm and humid conditions found in British houses. We tend to insulate our houses and to draughtproof them in order to cut down our heating bills, and the reduced level of ventilation which results produces ideal conditions for the mites to multiply. They especially like the insides of mattresses, pillows and soft furnishings, and also thrive inside children's cuddly toys.

It is not the mites themselves that cause allergies, but their faecal particles (droppings), which can set off the allergic process. These faecal particles are approximately the same size as pollen grains, and can become airborne for considerable periods of time, during which time they can be inhaled. Increased exposure to the house dust mite may be responsible for at least some of the increase that we have seen over the past 20 years in the number of people suffering from asthma, eczema and perennial allergic rhinitis. We know that between 70% and 80% of asthma and rhinitis sufferers are allergic to the house dust mite, which makes it a major trigger factor.

Ways of reducing the amount of house dust mites in the home, including discussion of the sprays you mention, are explored in Chapter 9.

I have asthma, which my doctor says is caused by stress. Does stress encourage the development of allergies?

There is little doubt that how we feel can influence our health, although this is not the same as saying that an illness or disorder is caused by stress. I suspect that your doctor meant that stress might trigger your asthma attacks. Emotional factors can trigger attacks in people with asthma, and therefore asthma can be more apparent in a person suffering high stress levels. However, the asthma has not been caused in the first place by stress, and it is not more common in people leading stressful lives (there is more information about the causes of asthma in Chapter 2).

What is true of asthma is also true of other allergies. Stress does not cause them, but it can trigger them, and certainly makes it more difficult to cope with the symptoms.

Inheritance

Why have I developed allergies when my sister hasn't?

Allergies occur because of a mixture of inherited and environmental factors. You were born with a predisposition to having allergies which you inherited from your parents. This is called atopy, and is discussed in more detail in the section called *Allergy explained* at the beginning of this chapter. Exactly which genes we inherit from our parents is largely a matter of chance, so you may have inherited more 'allergy genes' than your sister.

Given that you have this genetically determined tendency to develop allergies, then environmental factors become important. The way in which you are first exposed to various allergens will determine whether or not you develop allergic problems. If atopic people were never exposed to allergens, they would not develop allergies! The younger you are when you are first exposed to allergens and the greater the amount of allergen you encounter, the more likely you are to develop an allergy. For example, babies born just before or during the pollen season are more likely to develop hayfever and asthma than those born in winter.

Exposure to allergens is not the only important environmental factor. Interesting new evidence is suggesting that the more colds you catch in the first few years of life, the less likely you are to develop allergic disorders. We are also becoming more aware that there are other factors, called adjuvant factors, which can increase an individual's risk of developing allergies. These adjuvant factors include chemical air pollution and cigarette smoke. For example, babies born to mothers who smoke are twice as likely as other babies to develop asthma at some stage in their lives.

Once you have an allergy, there are a number of environmental factors, known as co-factors, which may – in some people – make that allergy more severe. These include exercise, aspirin, cold air, fevers and certain foodstuffs.

You can see that not all the children in an atopic family will go on to develop allergies. However, at the moment it is difficult to predict who will and who won't. Allergies, although more common in childhood and early adulthood, can develop at any time of life, even in old age, so your sister can't yet be certain that she has escaped completely.

Both of my children had eczema as small babies, developed asthma at around 4 years old, and started getting hayfever in their teens. Are all these problems related, why don't they all start at the same time, and has one caused the others?

The three problems you describe are related in that they are all allergic disorders which occur in atopic people, and they seem to be linked together in the way in which they are inherited. Some individuals (like your children) suffer from all three, others from just one or two.

No one really understands why it is that eczema occurs most commonly in babies, why asthma can appear at any age but does so most commonly in childhood, nor why hayfever is uncommon before a child is 10 years old (the incidence of these allergic disorders is shown in Figure 1). However, doctors often see this pattern of eczema being followed by asthma and then hayfever. An infant with eczema has a 50% chance of developing another form of allergic disorder before the age of 10 years. One problem does not cause the other as such (although untreated hayfever can make asthma worse) but they are three related conditions which can occur in the same individual.

Your question underlines the limitations of our current knowledge about exactly why particular allergies affect particular people at particular times in their lives. Scientists are

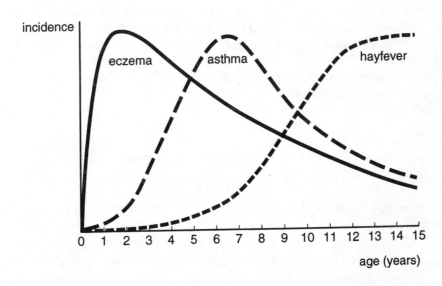

Figure 1: Incidence of eczema, asthma and hayfever at different ages.

currently trying to identify the genes on the chromosomes which cause people to inherit the tendency to develop allergies (genes determine the characteristics that we inherit from our parents, and chromosomes are the structures in our body cells that carry the genes). In the future this genetic research may provide a more specific answer to your questions.

The scale of the problem

When I was at school we had never heard of allergy. Now almost every child in my son's class seems to have asthma or an allergy of some kind. Are allergies more common these days?

It is not easy to know exactly how many people suffer from allergies because many of them never go to their doctor with their problem. Because of this, it is difficult to tell whether or not allergies really are becoming more common. However, there have been a small number of careful research studies into the prevalence of allergy (the number of people in the population suffering from allergic problems at any one time). These studies have been carried out over a number of years, and have shown fairly conclusively that allergies are becoming more common. Certainly most people's experience would seem, like your own, to agree with this.

Exactly how common are allergic problems?

This is a difficult question to answer, as a large number of people with allergies are never identified and many people who do know that they suffer from allergies never go to their doctors for help because they think their symptoms are too trivial. It is therefore difficult to estimate the true figure, but it is thought that as many as one in three people suffer from an allergy of some kind. It is becoming unusual to find a household where there is not at least one person who suffers from allergic problems.

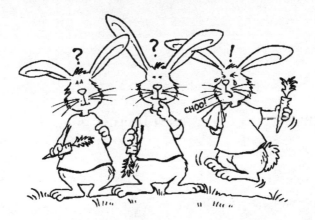

Almost everyone seems to have an allergy now. What are the most common diseases caused by allergy?

Allergy to plant pollens causing hayfever or seasonal allergic rhinitis (rhinitis is inflammation of the lining of the nose) is probably the most common allergy, affecting about 30% of the population. Asthma is becoming increasingly common, and currently about 15% of all children and 10% of adults are affected.

I know that hayfever is a problem caused by being allergic to pollen, but what other conditions are associated with allergy?

Quite a few different medical problems are at least partly caused by allergy, and these include asthma, hayfever, food allergies, drug allergies, eczema, dermatitis, urticaria (hives and nettle rash), angioedema and anaphylaxis. These are all discussed in other chapters of this book.

2
Asthma

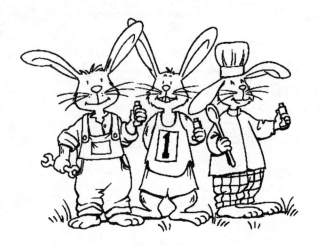

Introduction

Asthma is not new: it was described by the Chinese before 1000 BC, and was well known to the ancient Greeks. What is new is how asthma appears to be becoming more common, as over the past 50 years it has become one of the most important health problems in the Western world. In the United Kingdom almost 3 million people suffer from asthma, which means that at least one adult in every 10 has asthma, and at least one in every

7 children. Asthma is now the commonest chronic childhood medical condition, causing more school days to be lost than any other illness. The cost to the economy is enormous: it has been estimated that the annual financial burden of asthma to the National Health Service, the Department of Social Security and employers is in excess of £750,000,000.

As asthma is now so common and modern medicine so advanced, you might think that its diagnosis and treatment would be easy. Unfortunately this is not so. The symptoms of asthma can be very variable, and asthma can show itself in a number of different ways. It is not an exaggeration to say that everyone who has asthma is unique. Asthma symptoms can vary not just between individuals, but also in the same person on different occasions. This is, in part, because there are so many factors which can bring on the symptoms of asthma, and each factor can produce a different result. This is why it is so important to understand the whys and wherefores of your asthma, and to learn not just how to treat your symptoms but how to prevent them. With this knowledge will come the confidence that you can manage your asthma, which in turn should lead to a greater enjoyment of life.

Asthma explained

I have asthma, but no one has ever had the time to tell me exactly what is going on inside my lungs or why I sometimes have difficulty breathing. Please could you explain it to me?

As you know from your own experience, asthma is a condition in which it is difficult to move air in and out of your lungs as you breathe. This happens because your airways (the tubes inside your lungs, also called the bronchi) are narrowed. The underlying problem behind all this is that your airways are inflamed, that is they are irritated, swollen, red and sore. There are three main reasons why inflammation causes your airways to become narrowed.

- The inflamed airways are swollen and this makes the air passages narrower.
- The inflamed airways produce more mucus or phlegm, which adds to the obstruction.
- The inflamed airways are also irritable, and this make the muscles around them twitchy and more likely to go into spasm.

The airways of people with asthma are always slightly inflamed even when they otherwise feel well, which is why it is easy for various trigger factors such as exercise or colds to set off an asthma attack. There is a section on **Triggers** later in this chapter.

What caused my asthma?

When we think about the causes of asthma, we need to think about two things: what it was which made you develop asthma in the first place and, once asthma is established, what factors can set it off.

The reason why you developed asthma in the first place is because you come from a family which has a tendency to develop allergies. This inherited tendency to allergies is called atopy, and is discussed in more detail in the section on **Allergy explained** in Chapter 1. Asthma does seem to be – at least in part – an inherited condition. Having inherited this tendency, something then happened to you that turned the unseen tendency into actual asthma, and you will find some suggestions as to what this 'something' might have been in the answer to the next question in this section.

The factors which can set off your symptoms or cause you to have an acute asthma attack are usually referred to as 'triggers'. Your own triggers will be unique to you, but the more common ones are discussed in the section on **Triggers** later in this chapter. It is worth trying to find out what your triggers are, as some of them may be things which you can avoid, and that way you may be able to reduce your day-to-day symptoms and even limit the number of asthma attacks you have.

Why does asthma start?

Asthma is a condition which has lots of different causes, and each person's asthma is due to of a mixture of these causes. They can be divided up into hereditary and environmental factors, that is into what you have inherited from your parents and what is going on in the world around you.

We know that a predisposition to having asthma is inherited, so it is a condition which often runs in families. Scientists are currently trying to locate the gene on our chromosomes which passes on this asthma tendency from one generation to another (genes determine the characteristics that we inherit from our parents, and chromosomes are the structures in our body cells that carry the genes). In the long term, this research may help us to develop a cure for asthma.

The environmental factors which cause the tendency in a particular individual to become unmasked are difficult to identify. However, we know that if a young baby, or even the foetus before it is born, is exposed to high levels of certain substances to which people can be allergic (eg pollen or the house dust mite), then it is more likely that the child will develop asthma later in life. Certain things that happened after you were born may have made your inherited tendency more likely to develop into actual asthma, and these include:

* being brought up in a house where there was a pet, especially a cat;
* if you developed certain respiratory infections early in life;
* if foods such as cow's milk and eggs were introduced into your diet at an early age; or
* if you were born at a time of year when the pollen count was high.

We are becoming more aware that there are certain factors called adjuvant factors which can also increase your chances of getting asthma. These adjuvant factors include chemical air pollution and cigarette smoke. Babies born to mothers who smoke are twice as likely as other babies to develop asthma at some stage in their lives.

All these different factors help to explain why it is that you have developed asthma, but perhaps your brothers and sisters have not. It is not just a simple matter of inheritance, and it can be a difficult task to predict which family members will develop it – one which is made more difficult because there is no fixed age at which asthma starts. Although two-thirds of people with asthma first get their symptoms in childhood, it can develop at any time of life, even when people are in their sixties or seventies.

Why don't I have asthma all of the time?

Asthma varies a great deal from day to day and also over longer periods of time. You may have periods of your life lasting many years when your asthma is virtually trouble free. Similarly, you might find that even when your asthma is causing you problems, you have good days and bad days, or even good weeks and bad weeks.

Some of this variation can be explained. For example, on the one hand you may find that your asthma is less troublesome when you are on holiday and less stressed; on the other you may find that there are particular times of the year when your asthma is worse because of allergy to a particular type of pollen or changes in the weather. Some people's asthma is much worse when they have a cold, and better in between colds.

Another reason why asthma can be so variable is related to treatment. When you take the appropriate treatment regularly, your asthma symptoms should be well controlled, but if your treatment is either unsuitable for you or not taken regularly then it is going to be less effective.

Sometimes there is no obvious reason for the variations in your asthma symptoms. They just happen.

Why is asthma getting so much more common?

Asthma is certainly getting more common. Even when you take into account the fact that both doctors and the public are more aware of asthma as a condition (which means that milder cases which in the past might have been ignored are being correctly diagnosed), there is no doubt that the number of people with asthma has been increasing steadily over the last 30 years.

It is unlikely that there has been a major change in the way in which asthma is inherited during this relatively short time, and so we suspect that the reason for the increase is something to do with our environment. Increasing levels of air pollution, our modern diet with its high level of processed foods, our centrally-heated, double-glazed buildings with their high levels of house dust mite, and many other things about our modern day lifestyle might be responsible. There is a great deal of research being carried out at present on this subject, as asthma imposes a major social and financial burden upon most countries of the world.

Are there any differences between asthma in males and in females?

Although the different roles of men and women in our society are rapidly changing, it is still true that men are more likely to work outside of the home, and women within it. Therefore the different triggers for asthma that men and women encounter are likely to vary according to their environment. There are other differences: men are more likely to deny their asthma, and to be reluctant to seek diagnosis and treatment. Women may experience additional problems with their asthma during their menstrual periods. Other lifestyle factors such as smoking habits, participation in sport, and exposure to certain chemicals vary between the sexes.

There also seems to be a difference between males and females in the way that asthma behaves throughout life. In children under the age of seven, asthma is almost twice as common in boys as it is in girls. This appears to be because boy babies, although on average heavier and longer than girl babies, are born with smaller airways, which are more at risk of being affected by asthma. As boy children grow older, their airways become larger and they are more likely than girls to 'grow out of' their asthma and to become symptom-free. By the late teens, asthma is equally common in both sexes and by the twenties it is slightly more common in women and remains so throughout the later years.

I'm fed up with having to take medications every day. Can't asthma be cured?

No, it cannot be cured at present, although quite a large number of people with asthma seem to have symptom-free periods at some stage in their lives. Unfortunately they cannot be said to have been cured, as the symptoms often come back again. It seems that once you have asthma it is for life.

The aim of your asthma treatment is to enable you to make your life as normal as possible. Although this isn't the same as a cure, if your asthma is treated correctly it shouldn't be a major inconvenience. As you find your treatment so difficult to take, I suggest that you talk to your doctor and ask if there are ways in which it can be simplified.

Symptoms

My daughter and I both have asthma, but you would hardly know we had the same problem as our symptoms are so different. Is this unusual?

Not at all! Everyone who has asthma is unique, with each person having their own pattern and type of symptoms, and a different set of trigger factors (there is a section on *Triggers* later in this chapter). Although health care professionals can be expert in their knowledge of asthma in general, you are your own expert on your particular type of asthma. The more aware and better informed you are about it, the better you will be able to control your symptoms.

What are the typical symptoms of asthma?

It's not easy to answer this question, as there are many different ways in which asthma can show itself, and it can even be different in the same person at different times. The symptoms which occur most commonly are those of wheeze, cough and shortness of breath. These are often worse at night time and first thing on waking in the morning. Some doctors used to believe that people could only be diagnosed as having asthma if they wheezed, but we now realise that sometimes cough is the main symptom, especially in children.

As well as different symptoms there can be different patterns of asthma. Some people with asthma have symptoms almost every day; others have their symptoms in the form of acute attacks, and are well in between attacks.

I sometimes find it hard to judge how bad my asthma is. What symptoms mean I'm having a bad attack?

Obviously I don't know the details of your asthma and the problems it causes you, so I have to answer this question in general terms. Because of the wide variation in asthma symptoms in different people, it can be very difficult to decide how bad a particular attack is: what is bad for one person might be regarded as relatively mild by another. Bearing all that in mind, these are the warning signs which should warn you that an attack is a severe one.

- Symptoms which are unusually severe or unusually prolonged for you.
- Unusual symptoms which you have not had before.
- Breathlessness which is so bad that you find it hard to use your normal inhalers properly.
- Breathlessness which is so bad that you find it difficult to speak.
- Symptoms which are not relieved by your usual reliever medication.
- Only short lived (less than 4 hours) improvement from your usual reliever medication.
- A very fast heart rate (this can be felt at the wrist or at the neck), ie more than 120 beats per minute in an adult and more than 140 beats per minute in a child.
- A drop in your peak flow measurements to less than half of your usual level (peak flow measurements are discussed in the section on *Diagnosis and assessment* later in this chapter).
- Feeling exhausted by the effort to breathe.
- Any degree of blueness around your lips or of your tongue.

Asthma attacks can come on at any time. Mild attacks can develop into severe ones, and this can take anything from just a few minutes to several days. Asthma does not conform to a set pattern, and so it is therefore important to regard any worsening of your symptoms as being important. Always carry your reliever medication with you, use it when you feel your symptoms coming on, and consult your doctor if your reliever treatment does not produce a consistent improvement or if you are having to use it more often than is usual for you.

Triggers

What does my doctor mean when he talks about triggers of my asthma?

A trigger is anything which starts off a worsening of your asthma, that is it brings on your symptoms or an asthma attack. Not all people with asthma are troubled by the same trigger factors, and so something which causes you frequent problems might have no effect on someone else. The most common triggers are as follows.

- **Common cold virus (upper respiratory tract infections)**
  Most people's asthma gets worse when they develop a cold. This is particularly true in children, for whom this might be the only trigger. Often the symptoms of asthma persist after the cold itself has gone, sometimes for as long as six weeks.

- **Allergens**
  Exposure to allergens such as cat or dog fur, house dust mites, pollen and mould spores is a frequent cause of asthma attacks. People with asthma are particularly troubled by these allergens when they also have a cold.

- **Exercise**
  Coughing and wheezing brought on by exercise are very common among people with asthma. Exercise can be a particularly potent trigger factor when the air is cold and dry.

- **Emotion**
  Laughing, crying, getting excited or being upset can all trigger an asthma attack. This is particularly so in small children.

- **Cold air**
  Changes in air temperature, particularly going from warm into cold air, can bring on symptoms.

- **Air pollution**
  Traffic fumes, industrial waste products and cigarette smoke can all be important triggers for asthma.

- **Occupational triggers**
  Substances which are encountered in the work environment can become triggers for asthma if you develop an allergy to them.

- **Drugs**
  Certain drugs can trigger asthma attacks in some people. The commonest of these are aspirin, anti-inflammatory painkillers such as ibuprofen (brand names include Brufen, Nurofen and Cuprofen), and the beta-blocker drugs used for the treatment of high blood pressure. Once a problem with any of these drugs has been diagnosed, the drug in question should always be avoided as there are alternatives which are just as effective.

- **Foods**
  It is a common misconception that foodstuffs such as milk products or preservatives are frequent triggers for asthma. In fact it is relatively unusual for them to have this effect. There is no doubt that food allergies exist, but they tend to cause other allergic problems such as eczema or urticaria (both discussed in Chapter 3 on *Skin allergies*), and are rarely responsible for triggering asthma. Even if a food has been definitely identified as a trigger factor, it is important to remember that it is unlikely to be the only trigger involved. Although it would be sensible to avoid the food responsible wherever possible, you will probably need to use asthma medications as well to control your symptoms.

Why does other people's cigarette smoke make my asthma worse? I don't smoke myself.

Cigarette smoke is a complicated cocktail full of different chemicals and gases, many of which are very irritant to the lungs. Passive smoking (breathing in other people's cigarette smoke) can be irritating even to the lungs of people who do not have asthma, making them cough and feel tight-chested. In asthma the lungs are always inflamed, and are therefore more vulnerable to the effects of the smoke. It is likely to make you cough and wheeze, and the more inflamed your lungs are, the more chance there is that the smoke will aggravate your asthma.

My asthma seems to behave differently at different times of year, and I think this is to do with changes in the weather. Is this possible?

Yes, it is possible, as changes in the weather can affect your asthma in two ways. Firstly, changes in air temperature and humidity are both factors which can bring on asthma symptoms. This will be most noticeable when the air temperature changes from hot to cold, and when the air is either particularly dry or particularly wet and misty. Many people find that spring and autumn are the times when the weather seems to affect them the most.

Secondly, the weather affects the growth and the distribution of allergens that can trigger asthma, such as pollens, moulds and spores, and the house dust mite. The house dust mite and moulds enjoy warm, damp conditions, and are therefore likely to be particularly troublesome in the autumn. The pollen count (explained in the section on *Pollens* in Chapter 9) tends to be highest in the summer, on days on which the air is hot and still.

I have asthma and am keen not to do anything which might make it worse. Are there any sports or hobbies I should avoid because they could trigger my symptoms?

My aim in treating people with asthma is to adjust their medication so that, wherever possible, they are able to lead full lives and take part in all the activities that they find enjoyable. There are, however, certain activities which are more likely to bring on asthma than others.

Hobbies which involve fumes and dusts, such as model building and certain forms of DIY, might turn out to be triggers for your asthma. Any activity which brings you into contact with animals, especially ones with fur or hair, could also affect you.

When it comes to sports, it is worth remembering that many top rate athletes have asthma. Sport is less likely to bring on your symptoms if it is done in the warm (either in the summer or indoors), if the air is humid (such as in a swimming pool), if it is possible to perform warm-up exercises beforehand, and if the sport involves a steady level of activity. Sports which involve sudden bursts of vigorous exercise, especially if played outdoors in winter, might be more of a problem. However, if you find that you experience asthma symptoms because of exercise, these can be much reduced (or even abolished altogether) by taking two puffs of your reliever inhaler approximately 15 minutes before you start.

Exercise and contact with cats and horses all make my asthma worse. Can I make myself more resistant to these triggers?

Your general health is important in asthma. If you keep yourself fit, eat well, have enough sleep, and reduce the stress levels in your life as far as possible, then you are likely to be more resistant to the effects of your trigger factors. However, healthy living alone is unlikely to prevent all occurrences of your symptoms, and it is therefore vital that you take other measures to control your asthma.

Firstly you should reduce your exposure to things which are known to make the inflammation of your airways worse: for you these are cats and horses (Chapter 9 offers some suggestions for ways to avoid common allergens and other triggers). Don't try and avoid exercise, as there are ways in which you can exercise without becoming wheezy. Try taking two puffs of your reliever medication 10-15 minutes beforehand, and remember to warm up slowly with some gentle exercise before starting any more strenuous activity. Remember too that air pollution and cigarette smoke can make asthma worse.

The second most important way of reducing airways inflammation (the underlying problem in all asthma) is to use – on a regular basis – adequate levels of your preventer medications as prescribed by your doctor. Combining these two measures will make you less vulnerable to the numerous trigger factors, both known and as yet unknown, which can trigger the symptoms of your asthma.

I am 18 and have had asthma since I was 4 years old. Are there any particular jobs which I should avoid?

There are certain conditions which might be found in the workplace which are not advisable for anyone with asthma. Dust, fumes, smoke and chemicals are all triggers which are likely to make asthma worse, and should be avoided. Think carefully about what factors tend to trigger your asthma and try and avoid these as far as possible in your place of work. More and more employers are making their workplaces smoke-free zones, and I would thoroughly recommend anyone with asthma to try to work in an environment free of cigarette smoke (the reasons for this were discussed in an answer earlier in this section).

There are also certain jobs which you will not be allowed to do because you have asthma, either because they could affect your health (a firefighter cannot avoid triggers such as smoke and fumes, for example) or because other people could be put at risk if you had an asthma attack. These include deep sea diving and careers in the armed services, the Ambulance Service and the Fire Service. The Police Service assesses each applicant individually, and may accept candidates with a history of mild asthma in childhood but no current asthma.

My asthma has got a lot worse since I changed jobs. I know it's not stress-related, because I'm far more relaxed now than I was before in my previous work. Can you think of any other reasons why this has happened?

It is possible for a new job to exacerbate existing asthma or even to cause asthma in someone who has never had it before. As you already have asthma, you might now be more exposed at work to one or more of the trigger factors which make your asthma worse. For example you might have to work in a smoky office instead of a smoke-free one, or there might be high pollen levels in the area where you now work, or the nature of your work (eg if you are a school teacher – or a doctor!) might mean that you are exposed to a large number of other peoples' respiratory viruses.

There is also a type of asthma called occupational asthma

which is directly caused by exposure to particular substances found in some workplaces. These substances include:

- metals, including nickel, cobalt and aluminium;
- vegetable dusts such as coffee, grains and flour;
- animals and insects;
- polyurethane, spray paints and epoxy resins;
- soldering flux; and
- wood dusts.

This list is not exhaustive, but the Department of Health (address in Appendix 2) can supply more information about occupational triggers. Anyone who has developed asthma after starting a particular job and who suspects that a substance in the workplace may be responsible should ask to be referred to an occupational health specialist. The Health and Safety Executive (address also in Appendix 2) can help you, and you may be eligible for industrial compensation. It is important to decide whether you are suffering from occupational asthma as protecting you from the substance in question might make your asthma go away completely.

There is more information about occupational asthma and other workplace allergies in Chapter 7.

Diagnosis and assessment

How do doctors and nurses diagnose asthma if it can be so different in different people?

If you came to consult me, then the first very important step that I would take in making a diagnosis of asthma would be to spend as much time as possible in talking to you so that I was able to develop a clear picture about what symptoms you have, when they occur, what triggers them, and what makes them better. I would also want to ask you about other members of your family who have had problems with related atopic disorders: not only asthma, but also eczema, hayfever, perennial allergic rhinitis and urticaria (all these are discussed elsewhere in this book). There would be questions about your home and your work, to see if there were trigger factors there which might be important. I would then examine you, firstly to look specifically for clues to asthma (eg a change in the shape of your chest wall, wheezes in your chest, and whether you have eczema) and secondly to make sure that there was no suggestion of other problems which could be confused with asthma.

Usually by this stage it would be fairly clear whether or not you have asthma. However, it might still be useful for me to perform a number of different tests which would give me additional helpful information, even though they do not actually diagnose asthma. These tests include tests of how well your lungs are working (including peak flow measurement and more sophisticated lung function testing), skin prick testing for diagnosing allergies, and perhaps a blood test to look for evidence of allergy (all these tests are explained in detail in Appendix 1). In children I would measure height and weight so that I could assess their growth.

A particularly useful test can be to see what your response is to a dose of bronchodilator medication such as salbutamol (brand names include Ventolin and Aerolin) which will open up your airways if they are tight because of asthma. It is a very simple test which uses a small device called a peak flow meter (there is more about these meters later in this section). Using the meter I would measure how hard you can blow out first before, and then 15 minutes after, a dose of salbutamol. If you have asthma, an improvement of at least 15% should be seen. This improvement does not occur in people who do not have asthma, nor in people with chest problems due to other causes.

It might be that despite doing everything I have described, it would still not be possible to decide whether or not you have asthma. In this case, the best option would be to treat you with effective anti-asthma medication whilst monitoring your symptoms and peak flow recordings using a record card. If I saw a consistent improvement, you would almost certainly have asthma, and you would need to continue taking the treatment.

My son, aged 18 months, has a terrible cough, and my GP

says it is asthma and has prescribed some treatment. I thought asthma made you wheeze. How does he know this is asthma?

Asthma is different in every individual and different people experience a different combination of the common symptoms of wheeze, cough, shortness of breath and difficulty in breathing. In children, it is relatively common for asthma to produce coughing without wheezing. Your GP has probably asked you questions about your son's cough including, among many others, at what time of the day and night it is worse, and what triggers tend to bring it on. It is from this information that he would have made the diagnosis of asthma. If the cough is made better by the anti-asthma medications your GP has prescribed, then this is final proof that your son has asthma.

I think that my asthma has been brought on by being exposed to paint fumes at work. How do doctors diagnose occupational asthma?

To be able to diagnose you as having occupational asthma, two things are necessary. Firstly we would have to identify a particular chemical or allergen in your workplace which is known to cause occupational asthma. Certain paints and thinners fall into this category. Secondly we would have to demonstrate that your asthma is worse while you are working but better at weekends and during holidays taken away from your workplace. Monitoring your symptoms and lung function using a peak flow meter can help to do this. Final proof that your asthma is occupational can be obtained by protecting you from contact with the agent responsible and showing that your asthma has markedly improved.

There is more information about occupational asthma in Chapter 7 on *Allergies at work*.

I don't find it easy to tell how bad my asthma is. On days that I think I'm fine, my doctor says my chest is really tight. Is there a way that I can assess my asthma?

The simplest way of assessing your asthma is by noting how often your symptoms occur and how bad they are. This is often done with the help of a symptom score card or diary. By doing this, you will see when your symptoms occur, and you may be able to recognise a particular pattern (women may find their symptoms follow their menstrual cycle), or relate them to particular triggers such as colds or exposure to cigarette smoke. However, some people find that they are not very good at recognising their symptoms, and it sounds as if you may be one of these.

Another way of assessing your asthma is by measurement of your peak expiratory flow. This is a measurement of how hard you can blow, and is measured with the use of a small portable device called a peak flow meter (shown in Figure 2). Although there are charts which tell you what a 'normal' result is for someone of your age, sex and height, it is more useful to get a feel for your own personal normal level by making measurements when you are well. A reduction below this level in your peak flow recording tells you that your control of your asthma is not as good as it might be, and that you should either increase your treatment (if you have already agreed this with your doctor) or see your doctor as soon as possible.

My GP has given me a peak flow meter and has shown me how to blow into it, but I am not sure how often I should use it nor what to look out for. Can you help?

Peak flow meters are used to measure the amount of air that you can blow out from your lungs. In asthma, the flow from the lungs is reduced because of narrowing and tightness of the airways. Measuring your peak flow is therefore a way of measuring how

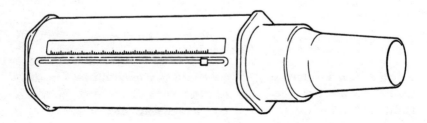

Figure 2: Peak flow meter.

much your asthma is affecting your lungs. The higher the recording, the better your lungs are functioning. Peak flow measurements vary from day to day a lot more in people with asthma than in people who do not have it. This variation becomes less once the asthma is properly treated, so it is a useful way of measuring the effectiveness of your treatment.

Different people find peak flow meters useful in different ways. Some like to measure their peak flow every day, as a check on how well their lungs are functioning. This can be particularly useful in people who have got so used to their symptoms that they sometimes fail to notice that their asthma is getting worse. A drop in their peak flow alerts them to the fact that they need to take action.

Others prefer to use their peak flow meters as tools to help them assess their asthma on the days when they are not feeling so good. On these days, measurement of peak flow can help to assess the severity of an attack, and can guide you in deciding what action to take.

Peak flow meters can also be used to assess how effective a change in treatment is. If your doctor suggests an alteration to your medication, you can monitor what benefits, if any, this brings by measuring your peak flow for a number of weeks after the change is made. If the change is effective, you will see a gradual increase in your peak flow over this time. The level of your peak flow will increase, and your peak flow recordings are also likely to become less variable.

In your case, I don't know how long you have had asthma, nor how bad it is. However, I would suggest that you might find it useful to measure your peak flow morning and evening on a daily basis for a period of about a month, so that you get a feel for what your 'normal' values are. You will probably find that your peak flow is slightly lower in the morning than in the evening. This variation, called diurnal variation, happens because your lungs are often a little tight on waking in the morning. This wears off during the day. Once you have a good idea of what your normal levels of peak flow are, you can use your peak flow meter as a way of assessing your lungs on days that you feel less than perfect.

Trouble signs to look out for are:

- if your peak flow recordings are dropping, or are below your normal level;
- if there is an increasing difference between your morning and your evening peak flow readings, with lower recordings in the mornings; and
- if there is an increasing variation between readings, with unusually low recordings on some days.

If you notice any of these, see your doctor as soon as possible, and consider increasing your treatment in the meantime.

Treatment

I am a teacher in a secondary school and I get very confused about all the different types of inhaler used by my pupils for their asthma. What's in all these different devices? Do they all work the same way?

Inhalers are the most efficient way of giving asthma medications, as it is better to take them by breathing them in rather than by swallowing them. They work more quickly when inhaled (because the drug is delivered directly to the lungs), and much smaller amounts of the drugs are needed to produce the same results, which in turn reduces the likelihood of side effects. However, small children are sometimes prescribed medications to take by mouth because they find inhalers difficult to use.

As you say, there are many different devices available (there is more information about them in the answer to the next question). This is because the different pharmaceutical companies make their own special devices designed to be used with the treatments they manufacture; some of these inhalers require more co-ordination to use them correctly than others. The particular medication and device which suits one child will not necessarily suit another – hence the range which you see among your pupils.

Broadly speaking, medications for the treatment of asthma can be divided into two groups which we call preventers and relievers. The colour of the inhaler will give you some idea of which type of drug it contains: preventer inhalers are usually brown, orange or maroon; reliever inhalers are usually blue; and long-acting reliever inhalers are usually green. This list is not complete, as other colours are used by some pharmaceutical companies, but you will find it useful as a rough guide.

Preventer medications reduce the degree of inflammation in the airways and are used, as the name implies, to prevent the symptoms of asthma and asthma attacks. These medications need to be used regularly even at times when there are no symptoms, and the dose can be adjusted according to need. Preventers do not work immediately, but instead act over a period of time to reduce inflammation and stabilise the asthma. They will have no effect in the case of an acute attack. Most preventers can be taken on a twice-daily basis and so most children will keep their preventer devices at home, but you may have a few pupils who need to take a dose of this type of medication during the school day.

Relievers relax and open up (dilate) the airways, and should only be used when symptoms occur. They should act quickly and effectively, relieving asthma symptoms after approximately 15 minutes. They have no long-term effect on asthma, as they do not reduce the amount of inflammation in the lungs. Children with asthma need free access to their reliever medication at all times as delay in taking these treatments could allow symptoms to develop into a severe asthma attack.

If you would like more information about how asthma affects children at school, then contact either the National Asthma Campaign or the National Asthma and Respiratory Training Centre (both addresses in Appendix 2) and ask for a schools information pack.

I'm not very happy with the inhalers I have for my asthma as I find it difficult to use them correctly. What can I do?

You don't say which type of inhaler you are using, but as you are finding it difficult to use, I suspect that it is a metered dose inhaler (shown in Figure 3). This is the most commonly-used type

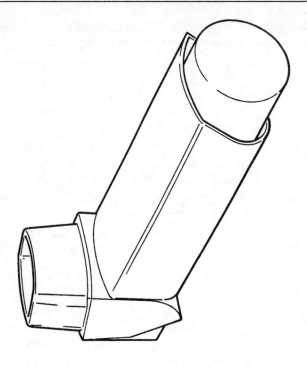

Figure 3: Metered dose inhaler.

of inhaler, and most asthma treatments are available in this form. However, it does have disadvantages, the most important one being that very good co-ordination is needed to use it properly.

I suggest that you go back to your GP's surgery or health centre, and talk to the person there who is responsible for asthma care. This may either be one of the doctors or a practice nurse, and you may find that they run a special asthma clinic. The answer to your problem may be some training in how to use your current inhaler correctly, or it may turn out that you would be better off with a different type of inhaler altogether.

Many different types of inhaler are now available (at least a dozen), and these various devices all have their own advantages and disadvantages. What suits one person will not suit another, and your doctor or nurse will be able to help you choose the one which suits you best and to show you how to use it. The following descriptions will give you some idea of the range available.

- The Volumatic (shown in Figure 4) is an example of a spacer device which fits on to a metered dose inhaler. The advantage of spacer devices are that they make the metered dose inhaler easy to use because there is no need to co-ordinate the firing of your inhaler with your breathing, so more of the drug is delivered to the lungs (where it is most needed) rather than perhaps ending up in the mouth. A disadvantage is the size of the device: it is too big to fit easily into a pocket or handbag.

- The Autohaler (shown in Figure 5) is an example of a breath-actuated metered dose inhaler. It is easy to use, as it releases the drug automatically when you breathe in through the mouthpiece, and so, as the puff of medication is always released at the right time, it requires little co-ordination. It is about the same size as a metered dose inhaler, so it is convenient to carry. However, only the drugs made by the pharmaceutical company which makes the Autohaler can be

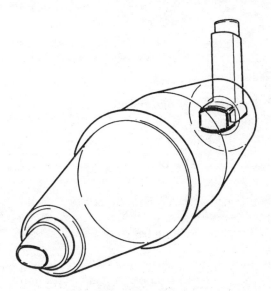

Figure 4: Volumatic.

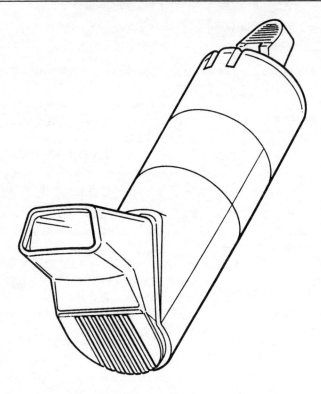

Figure 5: Autohaler.

used in it. If your particular asthma drugs are made by another company, you may have to choose a different device or switch to a different medication.

- The Diskhaler (shown in Figure 6) is an example of a dry powder device. In these devices the drugs are in powder form, rather than in the pressurised aerosol form used in metered dose inhalers, and some people find the taste of the powder form preferable. The Diskhaler is breath-actuated and therefore easy to use. Its particular advantage is that it is very easy to monitor exactly how many doses of the drug have been taken, something which is not possible with many of the other types of inhaler. A disadvantage is that the powder makes

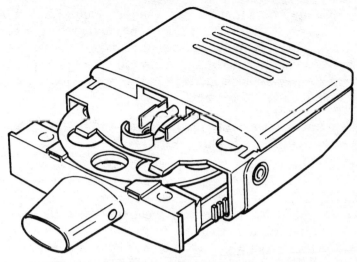

Figure 6: Diskhaler.

some people cough. Once again it can only be used with the drugs produced by the pharmaceutical company which manufactures it.

• The Turbohaler (shown in Figure 7) is another example of a breath-actuated dry powder device, and is one of the easiest of the inhalers to use correctly. An indicator shows you when it is

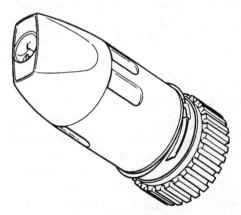

Figure 7: Turbohaler.

nearly empty, but otherwise you cannot monitor the number of doses taken. It will fit into a pocket or handbag. It can only be used with one particular reliever drug and one preventer, both made by the company which makes the device. The amount of powder in each dose is small, so it is less likely to cause coughing than the Diskhaler.

Can my lungs get used to my inhalers, and will they become less effective if I take them regularly?

Your inhalers are likely to be of two different types: a preventer and a reliever. You are meant to take your preventer inhaler regularly, and it won't work unless you do. There is no chance that your body will get used to this treatment – in fact, rather than needing to take more as time goes by, you may well find that you can take less as your asthma will come under better control. Nor will you become addicted to these inhalers, although you will probably need to continue to use them as at the moment we have no cure for asthma.

Your reliever inhaler should only be taken when you need it, which means when you actually have symptoms. If you take it in this way, it will continue to be effective. If you find that you are needing to use more than 3-4 doses a week of your reliever inhaler, then this is a sign that you are probably not taking enough of your preventer inhaler and that the dose of this needs to be adjusted. In this case you should consult your GP.

If you have an acute attack of asthma and find that your reliever inhaler is not having any effect, then this is a danger signal which tells you that the attack is a severe one, and that you should seek immediate medical help.

Which should I use first, my reliever or my preventer inhaler?

You will not often want to take both of these inhalers at the same time, as you should only take your reliever inhaler when you actually need to, which is when you have symptoms. Current thinking suggests that it may actually be harmful to use your reliever inhaler when you have no symptoms. If you do need to take both inhalers at the same time, it makes sense to use your reliever medication first, as it will open up your airways and let your preventer medication get deeper down into your lungs.

How do asthma treatments for young children or infants differ from those for adults?

Most of the treatments which are used for adults are also effective in children, and you will find that many children are on just the same medications as older people, often in the same doses and using the same types of inhalers. However there are certain medications which seem to work better in childhood, and also some which are not often used.

In children under one year of age, the commonly-prescribed reliever salbutamol (brand names include Ventolin and Aerolin) may not be effective, so a different type of bronchodilator drug called ipatropium (brand name Atrovent) is often preferred. Oral antihistamine medications such as ketotifen (Zaditen) seem to be much more effective in this age group than in adults, perhaps because allergens are more important triggers for asthma in early life. Sometimes it is necessary for people with asthma to take a corticosteroid medication such as prednisolone, a powerful drug which fights inflammation and allows the airway walls to recover. These corticosteroid drugs are not the same as the steroids misused by some athletes: those are anabolic steroids. If given in short courses of 3-7 days, corticosteroids are not harmful, but doctors try to avoid using them over long periods in childhood as they can have harmful side effects on growth and on bone strength. You will find more information about all these types of drugs elsewhere in this chapter.

The major challenge in treating very young children with asthma is not so much the choice of medication but how to deliver it efficiently to their lungs. More and more spacer devices are being developed which are especially designed for use with babies and very young children, and with the help of one of these it is now possible to use a metered dose inhaler (shown in Figure 3) to give asthma treatments to a child of any age. Children old enough to have developed sufficient co-ordination to use an inhaler by itself have the same choice of devices as adults (the range of inhalers available was discussed earlier in this section).

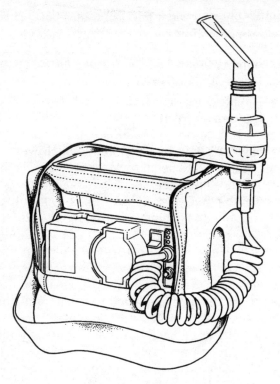

Figure 8: Nebuliser.

Nebulisers (an example is shown in Figure 8) are used more frequently in childhood than by adults – mainly because their use requires little co-operation from the child. They are machines which turn liquid medication into a fine mist which can then be inhaled. Adults usually only need to use a nebuliser if they have very severe asthma, or are unable for some reason (eg arthritis in the hands) to manage ordinary inhaler devices.

My asthma can be very variable, and my doctor often asks me to increase or decrease the number of puffs of my preventer inhaler. He's done this so often that I feel I know as well, if not better than him, how much I need. Can I adjust the dose of medication myself?

You are right: sometimes the person with asthma is the one who knows best how good or bad the asthma is at any particular time. However, it is not a good idea to make all the changes to your treatment yourself. If you did, your doctor would never know what dose you were taking or how you were feeling, and there is always the chance that you might get it wrong and take either too much or – more dangerously – too little of your treatment.

A very good and effective compromise would be to agree on a plan of self-management with your doctor. The simplest self-management plan is just to arrange to see your doctor or your practice asthma nurse when your symptoms get worse. More comprehensive plans are based on your peak flow measurements (explained in the previous section on *Diagnosis and assessment*) and the action you will take in altering your medication will depend on changes in your peak flow when compared to your own normal level. I suggest that you discuss this with your doctor, and ask him if he would be willing to write a self-management plan with you which you could use to take more responsibility for your treatment yourself.

My 9-year-old son has been diagnosed as having asthma, and I am worried about the inhalers our doctor has put him on. Are the side effects of asthma treatments dangerous?

Before you start worrying too much about the side effects of drug treatments for asthma, please remember that asthma itself can be dangerous. In children, poorly-controlled asthma can cause chest deformities, poor growth, and a reduction in academic performance because of lost sleep and lost time at school, as well as a decrease in the quality of life for the whole family. In adults, asthma can be a life-threatening condition, although it is relatively rare for anyone to die from it. It is therefore important to view the side effects of asthma treatment from within this perspective.

Side effects – if any – will depend upon which treatments your son is taking. Any side effects his reliever medications might have will be temporary, lasting for a maximum of four hours after he takes the drug. There are two main types of reliever, and they have different side effects.

- The first group, which includes salbutamol (Aerolin, Ventolin) and terbutaline (Bricanyl), can cause a fine trembling, particularly noticeable in the hands. If a large dose of these medications is taken, the heart rate may increase. This does not damage the heart, but may feel uncomfortable.
- The second group, which includes ipatropium (Atrovent) and oxitropium (Oxivent) can cause a dry mouth and blurred vision. Occasionally difficulty in passing urine and constipation can occur.

There is much more concern these days about the side effects of the preventer medications. If your son is taking sodium cromoglycate (Intal) you need not worry, as this drug has no side effects of any kind. If he has been prescribed an inhaled steroid such as beclomethasone (Aerobec, Becotide) or budesonide (Pulmicort), then again you need not be concerned providing your son is taking a low dose. (Discuss the dose with your doctor, but as a general rule, a low dose is regarded as up to 400 micrograms a day). The only side effects that he may experience are hoarseness and oral thrush, a fungal infection which may show up as a red rash with white spots in the mouth and on the back of the throat. Both of these side effects can be prevented by using a spacer device (an example was shown in Figure 4) which will reduce the amount of medication which is left in the mouth by increasing the delivery to the lungs.

At higher doses, inhaled steroids may cause children's growth to slow down temporarily. In adults there may be a risk of thinning of the bones (osteoporosis). These risks are particularly high if oral steroid tablets such as prednisolone are taken for long periods (months or years). Short courses of prednisolone tablets (ie for less than two weeks) taken up to four times a year are not thought to cause significant side effects. If your son has to take steroid tablets regularly and you are concerned about their side effects, then talk it over with your doctor. Whatever you do, do not stop treatment with steroid tablets suddenly: this can be very dangerous. (Incidentally, the steroids that are used in asthma medications are not the same as those abused by some athletes.

Those are anabolic steroids; the ones used for asthma are a different type called corticosteroids.)

Listed together like this, all these side effects sound rather alarming, but all these risks must be balanced against the risks of uncontrolled asthma. Drugs such as Becotide have been in use for over 20 years, and have an extremely good track record for safety. People who have been using inhaled steroid medications over a long period of time during their childhood are no shorter than their friends who do not have asthma, and are probably considerably taller than they would have been had their asthma remained untreated.

The safest course of action is for your son to take adequate treatment with effective preventer medications, preferably by the inhaled route, with the aim of gaining control of his asthma, and then to reduce his preventer treatment to the lowest dose which keeps his asthma well controlled. He should then use his reliever inhaler only when he has symptoms.

I have just discovered that I am pregnant, and I am worried that my asthma treatment could be harmful to my baby. Should I stop my inhalers?

I can understand your concern, but there is no need for you to stop your inhalers. Even if you are using a steroid preventer inhaler, the dose will not be large enough to pose any threat to your baby's well-being (the side effects of steroid inhalers were discussed in the answer to the previous question). What might be more likely to cause your baby a problem would be if your asthma were to get worse. My advice is that you continue using your inhalers, adjusting them as necessary under your GP's supervision so that your asthma is kept under the best possible control.

I have heard that all asthma inhalers contain CFCs which harm the environment. Is this true and, if so, what can I do about it other than to stop using my inhalers?

Please don't stop using your asthma treatment: this will do you a lot of harm and do absolutely nothing to help the environment! You don't need to worry about the effect of the CFCs (chlorofluorocarbons) in your inhalers, as the manufacturers are being forced to address this issue. As all asthma inhalers will have to be CFC-free by 1999, the manufacturers are rapidly developing inhalers made with gases not thought to be harmful to the atmosphere. These changes should not alter the effectiveness of your treatments.

My friend, who lives in France, is receiving desensitization treatment for her asthma. My GP won't perform this treatment for me. Why not?

Doctors have a number of concerns about desensitization treatment (also called immunotherapy), the most important of which is safety. Sometimes people undergoing this treatment can suffer a severe, even life-threatening, allergic reaction. Because of this, these treatments should only be given in specialist centres which have experience of both administering this type of treatment and of treating any untoward reactions.

We also have concerns about the usefulness of this type of treatment. There is little evidence to show that allergen desensitization has much of a beneficial effect upon asthma, as asthma is not usually triggered by just one allergen but by a large number of different factors. Allergen desensitization needs to be a lifelong treatment, so in view of this and its other drawbacks, it is not a form of treatment that we recommend for asthma, although it is still used in severe allergic reactions and anaphylaxis, and occasionally in hayfever.

There is more information about desensitization in the section on *Allergy explained* in Chapter 1, and on its use in anaphylaxis in the section on *Living with anaphylaxis* in Chapter 6.

My husband, who has asthma, is very overweight. Would his asthma get better if he lost weight?

Almost certainly. His lungs and heart are currently having to work much harder than they ought to supply his body with oxygen, and this is bound to be making his asthma worse. If he lost weight, not only would his asthma be likely to improve, but he might also feel fitter and healthier in lots of other ways as well.

Asthma and allergy

Is all asthma allergic?

Doctors used to describe asthma as being either extrinsic, meaning that it was triggered by external factors such as allergens, or intrinsic, meaning that it was not associated with allergy. It is now clear that things are not that simple and that there is a great deal of overlap between them. Most people with asthma are vulnerable to external triggers, but to a varying degree depending on the individual. As a general rule, the younger you were when you developed your asthma, the more closely it will be linked to allergy. People who develop asthma at a later age seem to have more persistent symptoms which are not so clearly linked to triggers such as allergens, upper respiratory tract infections (colds) or atmospheric conditions.

I was tested recently with skin prick tests and these showed that I have several allergies as well as asthma. Are there treatments I can use to help these allergies?

When you know that you are allergic to something, it is common sense to try and reduce your exposure to it, as it is likely to be making your asthma worse. There are some suggestions for ways of avoiding allergens in Chapter 9.

Unfortunately there are some allergens such as pollen which cannot be avoided completely. In this case an antihistamine medication may be a useful addition to your normal asthma treatment. It would be better for your GP to prescribe antihistamines for you (rather than you buying them over the counter from the chemist), as that way your doctor can be sure that you really need them and also give you one which is safe in combination with your other medications.

Antihistamines work by blocking the effects of histamine, the substance which is produced when an allergic reaction takes place (there is more information about this in the section on *Allergy explained* in Chapter 1). They are usually taken by mouth, and are available in both liquid and tablet form. The newer preparations cause less drowsiness than the old ones, and some only need to be taken once a day, which is much easier to remember.

My daughter has just been diagnosed as having asthma. We have a cat, whom we regard as a member of the family. Do I really have to get rid of him?

Ideally, no child with asthma should live in a home where there are dogs, cats or other furry animals. However, I do understand your dilemma, as pets are often much loved family members which their owners would be reluctant to lose. If your daughter's asthma is mild and is well controlled on the treatment prescribed by your doctor, then there is no need to do anything about your cat. If her asthma is difficult to control, and particularly if contact with the cat seems to make things worse, then you need to take measures to reduce her exposure to the cat's allergen. Your doctor should be able to advise you just how serious your daughter's asthma is, and how important a part any allergy to your cat is likely to be playing.

If the cat is a problem, then the most effective solution would be to find a new home for him, remembering that it can take up to six months for cleaning and vacuuming to remove all traces of cat hair and dander (a combination of the saliva which cats use for grooming and the scales from their hair or fur). There are also other moves you can try. Washing the cat once a week is said to

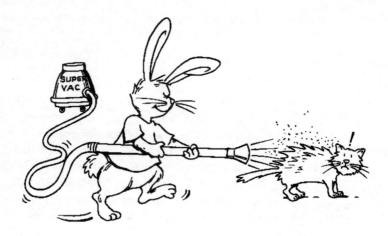

reduce the amount of allergen the cat spreads, but this is easier said than done. Ensuring that the cat does not go upstairs in the house and especially into your daughter's bedroom may improve things. However, the cat allergen is very potent, and even the small amount spread on the bottoms of shoes can be enough to be troublesome to someone with asthma.

I have asthma which is not too bad in the winter, but which can be much worse in spring and summer when I have trouble with hayfever. Why does my hayfever make things worse?

There are two main reasons why this happens. Firstly, your lungs may be affected by the same allergens as your nose, which would make it easy to understand why both problems get worse together. Secondly, even if your lungs are not vulnerable to these allergens, what is going on in your upper airway can affect your lower airway. Your nose is the top part of a continuous system which reaches down to the very bases of your lungs: if the upper part of this tube is inflamed, the inflammation can spread downwards into the lungs.

It is important to ensure that your hayfever is treated as successfully as possible – not just from the point of view of your nose, but also for the sake of your asthma. This might mean using both an anti-inflammatory nasal spray and an antihistamine preparation taken by mouth. Hayfever is discussed in detail in Chapter 4, and you will find more information about these treatments there.

I am sure that certain foods make my asthma worse. My doctor says that food allergies are not a cause of asthma. Can food allergies cause asthma?

Food allergies certainly exist (they are discussed in Chapter 5) but it is relatively unusual for them to be responsible for triggering asthma. They are only an important trigger in a very few people, and these people usually also have a strong tendency to allergies, in particular an allergic problem called urticaria (discussed in the section on *Skin allergies explained* in Chapter 3). The most likely foods to cause this type of problem are peanut, cow's milk, true nuts, seafood and shellfish. It is possible to test you for allergies to these foods, and you should discuss this with your doctor and ask to be referred to a specialist if necessary.

In any case, it is unlikely that a food allergy is the only trigger for your asthma. Even if you managed completely to avoid any foods to which you were proved to be allergic, you would probably still need to continue using your regular asthma medication.

What about food additives – are they a cause of asthma?

Food additives are blamed for a large number of medical conditions but in reality they cause relatively few. There are only two food additives which are known to bring on attacks of asthma.

- Tartrazine (E number 102) is a yellow colouring found in many sweets and soft drinks.
- Sodium metabisulphate is an antioxidant used to stop food going rancid. It is found in canned and dried foods, soft drinks and wine, and in packet soup, sauces and gravy mixes.

These two additives are clearly marked on food labels in the United Kingdom, and it would be advisable for people with asthma to avoid them.

There are a lot of allergic problems in my family. Will breast-feeding my baby make her less likely to develop asthma? How long should I continue for?

Bottle-fed babies are more likely to develop allergic conditions – including asthma – when compared to babies who are breast-fed. I would recommend that you breast-feed, providing that you are able to. You should continue for at least four months, as it is in these first months of life that babies are particularly prone to developing allergies.

Breast-feeding can have even more of a protective effect if the mother herself can avoid eating foods frequently associated with allergies during the period when she is breast-feeding. In practice this can be very difficult to do, as the culprits include common foods such as cow's milk, eggs and nuts. Unless your family has a very strong history of allergy, I would suggest that you eat a normal diet.

There is more information on breast-feeding and food allergies in Chapter 5.

I know that I am allergic to the house dust mite and that it affects my asthma. Is it worth me buying an ionizer or a dehumidifier?

There are a large number of devices on the market which claim to help people who have asthma. Among them are ionizers and dehumidifiers, both of which can reduce the amount of the house dust mite allergen circulating in the air. Ionizers do this by adding a negative electrical charge to particles in the air which encourages them to settle. Dehumidifiers work by reducing humidity and making conditions inside the house less favourable for the house dust mite.

Before you buy either of these (often expensive) devices, it is worth looking at the scientific evidence for their usefulness, as many of the manufacturers' claims are unfounded. Small changes in the amount of house dust mite circulating in the air will not necessarily be associated with an improvement in your asthma which, after all, is the result you are after. Other methods of decreasing house dust mite levels, as outlined in Chapter 9, are much more likely to be effective in reducing your symptoms.

Both my husband and I have asthma, and we are about to move house. Is there any type of house that might be particularly suitable for us?

By choosing your new house carefully you might be able to make quite a difference to your asthma, and I would suggest that you consider the following issues, which are discussed in more detail in Chapter 9.

- **Traffic pollution**
  Try and choose a house which is not on a main road and where it is not necessary for you to walk along busy roads, for example to get to the local shops or to the local school.

- **Pollens**
  If you are allergic to grass and tree pollen, it would be sensible to choose a house which is not surrounded by fields and which does not have a large collection of trees nearby (although pollens can travel long distances in the wind).

- **Animals and pets**
  If you are allergic to furry animals, you should avoid situations where you might find contact with animals difficult to avoid. As it can take many months of vigorous cleaning to remove animal hair and allergens from a home, it would be sensible to try to avoid buying a house where pets (particularly cats) have been kept.

- **Ventilation**
  In order to be energy efficient, modern houses tend to be tightly sealed with poor ventilation. Unfortunately, the less well ventilated the house, the higher the levels of the house dust mite inside it, because the house dust mite enjoys warm, humid conditions. It would be wise for you to consider purchasing an older style of house which has features such as fireplaces and air bricks which increase ventilation.

- **Flooring**
  Fitted carpets increase levels of dust and therefore of the house dust mite. Smooth floor surfaces such as lino, wood flooring or tiles are easier to keep clean and dust free.

- **Heating**
  Forms of heating which blow the air around (such as ducted hot air heating and underfloor heating) tend to aggravate asthma symptoms as they increase the amount of house dust mite allergen in the air. The least troublesome form of heating is gas central heating using radiators and with the gas boiler well away from the living area and the bedrooms.

3
Skin allergies

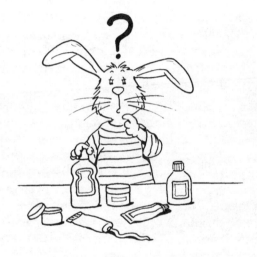

Introduction

The skin is the largest organ of the body. As it is the part of us which is in most direct contact with the rest of the world, it is not surprising that it is often affected by allergies. For example, between 10% and 12% of children and about 1% of adults have eczema.

It can be very difficult to work out whether your skin problem is due to an allergy and, if so, which allergen is responsible, as most people meet many different substances as part of their everyday lives. There are, however, a number of tests which a dermatologist (skin specialist) can use to identify the culprits. Once you know the culprits, you can take action to avoid coming into contact with them in the future. If this is not possible, then treatments are available which can help to relieve your symptoms.

Skin allergies explained

I have eczema, but recently I developed a different sort of skin rash as well, which my doctor told me was called urticaria. She said it wasn't a skin allergy as such, even though it affected my skin. What's the difference between skin allergies and urticaria?

Skin allergies (eczema and dermatitis) affect atopic people, that is people who have an inherited tendency to developing allergies (atopy is discussed in more detail in the section on *Allergy explained* in Chapter 1). They are always caused by allergens and they only affect the skin. Once established, they can be long-lasting: eczema can continue for months or even years.

Urticaria (also known as nettle rash or hives) can occur in both atopic and non-atopic people, and can be triggered by a wide range of stimuli, not all of which are allergens. In some cases of urticaria, especially when it is recurrent, the cause cannot be found, but probable causes include the following.

Allergic causes

- Allergens such as bee and wasp stings, foods such as milk, nuts, beans, fish and shellfish, and drugs such as penicillin.

Non-allergic causes

- Physical causes such as cold, heat, pressure, water and sunlight.
- Some drugs, such as ibuprofen (trade names include Brufen, Nurofen, Cuprofen), aspirin, paracetamol, and some drugs used in the treatment of arthritis.

- Some food dyes, such as tartrazine (E number 102), and some food preservatives such as ascorbic acid, sulphites and other antioxidants.
- Virus infections.

Urticaria affects the most superficial layers of the skin, and appears as multiple itchy lumps which are often red in colour. The rash lasts a relatively short time, usually disappearing within 24-72 hours. Although it affects the skin, it is often part of a more generalised allergic reaction which can affect other parts of the body including the eyes, nose, lungs and throat.

There is also another type of skin rash which can be caused by a generalised allergic reaction that affects other parts of the body as well. This is angioedema, which is a little like urticaria but, because it occurs in the deeper layers of the skin and the tissues beneath the skin, it causes larger swellings which are not itchy but can be painful.

Recently my doctor prescribed a course of antibiotics for a urinary infection I had, and the day after taking the first dose I was covered from head to toe in the most awful itchy rash. My doctor now tells me I am allergic to that antibiotic, and that I must avoid not only that one but a number of others too from now on. The trouble is that I am now scared that I will react to all antibiotics and I worry about what will happen if I need to take one in the future. Can I be tested with the other antibiotics to make sure they are safe?

Many different types of drugs can cause allergic reactions, but you are more likely to develop an allergy to a drug which you only take occasionally rather than to one you take continuously. Drugs which are injected or which are applied directly to the skin are more likely to provoke an allergic reaction than those which are taken by mouth and swallowed. Children and elderly people are less likely to develop drug allergies than adults because the immune system is less active at the extremes of age.

In your case you know that your allergic reaction was caused by an antibiotic. Together with anti-inflammatory painkilling drugs such as aspirin and ibuprofen (brand names include Brufen, Nurofen and Cuprofen), antibiotics are the most common cause of allergic problems. As many as one in 20 people react to the antibiotic amoxycillin, and trimethoprim can also cause allergic rashes. It is likely that it was one of these which was prescribed for your infection.

Allergic reactions to antibiotics are rarely dangerous, but the rash, which is a form of urticaria, can be itchy and uncomfortable. You correctly reported your allergic reaction to your GP, who will have made a note of it in your case records. As your reaction was quite unpleasant, your doctor will ensure that you are given a different type of antibiotic in the future. There are a number of different groups or families of antibiotics – amoxycillin is a form of penicillin, for example – and if you are allergic to one member of a group, you should assume that you are allergic to all thé members of that group.

It is very unlikely that you are allergic to more than one of the groups of antibiotics, so the ones which you must avoid from now on will all belong to the same family. Try not to worry about needing treatment in the future, as all the other antibiotics in the other families should be safe for you to take. As the cause of your rash was so obvious, I would not suggest that you need to be tested in any way.

I developed a rash about five days after starting a course of antibiotics. My doctor told me that it looked like a reaction to the antibiotic, and to avoid taking that drug in the future. I am not convinced, as the rash came on the day I finished the course of treatment. Could it really still have been caused by the drug?

Yes. If you have not taken a particular drug before, then the rash caused by an allergy to it can come on as late as two weeks after starting treatment with it – it can take that long for the initial allergic reaction to develop. However, if you had taken that drug in the past you would have already developed the allergy to it, and then the rash would start within a day of your treatment beginning (which is what usually happens – allergies do not happen the first time you are exposed to a particular allergen).

Your doctor thought that the rash looked typical of a drug reaction, and so I think you would be wise to assume that you are allergic to that particular antibiotic and to avoid it from now on.

A colleague at work sometimes has red, swollen hands. When we ask what's wrong, she says that it's just her dermatitis but doesn't explain any further. Could you please tell us what it is?

Dermatitis is the name given to an inflammatory reaction affecting the skin (the process of inflammation is explained in the section on *Symptoms* in Chapter 1). The inflammation causes swelling in both the superficial (surface) and deeper layers of the skin, and it can be caused by contact with a wide variety of substances. The name dermatitis comes from the Greek: 'derma' meaning 'skin', and '-itis' meaning 'inflammation'.

Dermatitis can be acute (sudden) or chronic (long-lasting). If it is acute, the skin is often red, swollen and tender, and may be itchy. In more chronic dermatitis the skin becomes thickened and may be scaly.

Dermatitis is caused by contact between the skin and an allergen, which accounts for its full medical name of allergic contact dermatitis. Because of this, it most commonly occurs on the hands and forearms, which are the parts of the body most likely to come into contact with potential allergens. It is important to realise that dermatitis can occur after contact with a substance that has been handled with no problem over a large number of years, as well as with substances to which the skin has just been exposed recently. We still don't know why the skin can suddenly be affected by something which it has tolerated happily for a long period of time.

A child at my son's school always seems to be itching and scratching because of eczema. Is eczema catching and should I keep my son away from this other boy?

There is no need for that, as eczema is not catching or infectious in any way. There are skin infections causing itching and scratching which are contagious, but eczema is not one of them.

Eczema is a form of dermatitis which happens in people who

are prone to developing allergies, which means they have an inherited tendency called atopy (atopy is discussed in detail in the section on *Allergy explained* in Chapter 1). This explains the other name for eczema, which is atopic dermatitis. It is a chronic (long-lasting) form of skin inflammation which tends to vary in severity over periods of time, getting worse and getting better for no apparent reason. It usually occurs for the first time in early childhood, although it can start at any time of life.

In mild cases of eczema, the skin is dry and scaly, but it can become red and weepy if the eczema is severe. It has a tendency to affect particular parts of the body, such as the wrists, the ankles, inside the elbows, and behind the knees and ears. Eczema irritates the skin and makes it itchy, which is why your son's friend keeps wanting to scratch.

You've just said that eczema is a form of dermatitis, so what's the difference between the two?

It can be confusing, and the confusion arises because of the way in which the word dermatitis is used. Because the word simply means 'inflammation of the skin' it can be correctly applied to a number of skin conditions, of which eczema (atopic dermatitis) is one. In practice it is most often used as a shorthand term for allergic contact dermatitis, and atopic dermatitis is referred to as eczema, which is what I have done in this book.

Eczema is a form of dermatitis in the broader sense of the word, ie it is a particular type of skin inflammation. It occurs in people who are atopic, which means they have an inherited tendency towards developing allergies. Eczema usually occurs in children born into families with a history of eczema, asthma or hayfever, and is often associated with dry skin. It usually begins before a child is 2 years old, and often before the age of 6 months. In a young infant it frequently starts on the trunk of the body and on the face, and as the child gets older the backs of the knees and the insides of the elbows become affected. It often improves with age, and in many children it disappears by the time they are 4 years old. However, it may become worse again later on in life, and about a quarter of all children with severe eczema will continue to have it into adult life.

Dermatitis – by which I mean allergic contact dermatitis – is unusual in children and in elderly people, becomes more common in adulthood, and occurs more often in females than in males. The allergens which most commonly cause allergic contact dermatitis are nickel, formaldehyde, and those found in plants and rubber products (these are all discussed in the section on *Dermatitis* later in this chapter). The parts of the body affected by dermatitis are limited to those which have come into contact with the allergen that has caused it.

Treatment for the two conditions also differs. The mainstay of treatment in eczema is the regular use of emollients (skin moisturising and softening creams) with the addition of steroid-containing creams when necessary. If the substance responsible for causing allergic contact dermatitis can be identified and avoided, then long-term treatment is unnecessary, although steroid creams and emollients may be needed for a time to clear the dermatitis up.

I get eczema but only on my hands. Why is this?

This could be eczema, but it seems more likely (for the reasons explained in the answer to the previous question) that your problem is due to a contact dermatitis. I think your hands are probably coming into contact with something to which they are vulnerable, and this is triggering your dermatitis.

You need to think carefully about what might be causing your dermatitis, and then try to avoid contact with it. For example, do you wear rubber gloves? These often contain latex, which can cause an allergic reaction. Do you use any chemicals at work? What about other allergens known to cause dermatitis (you will find a list of these in the section on *Dermatitis* later in this chapter)?

If you cannot identify what is causing your dermatitis, patch testing using a wide range of substances might come up with the answer. This is discussed in more detail in Appendix 1, and can be organised if your GP refers you to a dermatologist (skin specialist).

My baby has eczema. Does this mean that she is going to develop asthma or hayfever?

Asthma, eczema and hayfever are all linked, in that they are all atopic disorders caused by the same inherited predisposition (atopy is discussed in detail in the section on *Allergy explained* in Chapter 1). However, asthma and hayfever are not only due to heredity, as environmental factors also play a part. This means that although there is a much higher chance that a baby with eczema will go on to develop another of the atopic disorders, it is not inevitable, and so your daughter will not necessarily develop these other conditions.

Research is currently underway to see whether or not the use of certain antihistamine medications, given by mouth from as early as 4 weeks old, can reduce the risk of a baby who already has eczema developing asthma. The researchers are looking at babies from families where there is a history of allergies, because these babies have a greater chance of developing asthma. The antihistamines (called ketotifen and cetirizine) are currently used for the treatment of allergic disorders, but it would be an exciting prospect if they could also be used to prevent these problems from developing.

My baby developed eczema very early on – he was only 2 weeks old – and there is a lot of asthma and hayfever in my family. Does this mean he is less likely to grow out of his eczema?

As your son developed his eczema at such an early age, this probably means that he has a strong atopic tendency (atopy is discussed in detail in the section on *Allergy explained* in Chapter 1). Because of this, he is less likely to grow out of his eczema than a child who developed similar symptoms at a later age. But you shouldn't despair: only one out of every four children with severe eczema still have it by the time they are an adult, so the outlook really isn't that bad. The frustrating thing is that there is no way that we can predict whether your son will be one of the lucky ones or not.

Causes of eczema

My baby son has eczema. Why? What causes it?

The predisposition towards having eczema is something you inherit, similar to the way in which asthma is inherited, and because of this, it is a condition which often runs in families. Eczema is related to other atopic disorders, such as asthma and hayfever: they all result from the way in which you respond to an allergen by producing specific IgE allergy antibodies (this is discussed in more detail in the section on *Allergy explained* in Chapter 1). I would not be at all surprised to learn that either you or your baby's father have at least one of these allergic problems.

Having inherited this predisposition, a number of everyday factors might have increased your son's likelihood of developing eczema. For example, eggs and cow's milk might have been included in his diet at an early age, or there might be a pet (especially a cat) in the house, or good insulation and central heating might have led to high levels of the house dust mite. Once eczema becomes established, the skin is particularly vulnerable to a large number of materials including certain chemicals found in skin creams, some foods, and many washing powders: all of these can lead to flare ups of the eczema. Eczema is also made worse if the skin is damaged, perhaps by scratching, or because the skin has become too dry. If your son scratches, his skin will become more itchy, and a vicious circle will be built up in which he continually makes the condition of his skin worse.

Eczema can vary in severity from very mild to very severe. In mild cases, eczema may be the only allergy-related problem. At the other end of the spectrum, people with severe generalised eczema often also have asthma and hayfever.

Is there any way to prevent eczema?

Some research studies have shown that where allergies run in the family, breast-fed babies are less likely to develop eczema than bottle-fed babies. Eczema tends to start in infancy, and at this age food allergens (such as those found in eggs and cow's milk) are more important in the development of allergic disorders than those found in the air (such as the house dust mite and pollens). Because milk and egg proteins eaten by a mother are passed through into her breast milk, it may be that a breast-feeding mother should avoid these foods in her own diet to reduce the risk of eczema even more (although before doing this she should consult her doctor). However it makes sense to limit the exposure of small babies to ALL allergens as much as possible.

My child's eczema has suddenly got worse. What could be doing this?

Exposure to any of the factors which are responsible for the development of eczema can also make existing eczema worse. Examples include allergens such as the house dust mite, cat and dog fur, and pollens; chemicals such as lanolin, fragrances and detergents; and also factors such as low humidity, virus infections and stress. Everyone with eczema is different, and will be affected by different triggers. I suggest you consider the following things and see if any of them apply to your child. The list is not exhaustive, but it may help you to track down the specific cause.

- **Diet**
  Is there anything which your child has just started to eat (or has eaten a lot of) in the few days prior to the flare up?

- **Chemicals**
  Have you started using a new washing powder? Have you started using a different skin cream, soap or shampoo? Remember that occasionally manufacturers change the formulation of their products, so a product you have happily used in the past may suddenly become a problem.

- **Stress**
  Stress and anxiety can often make eczema worse.

- **Other allergens**
  Exposure to the house dust mite can precipitate eczema in some people. House dust mites love beds, soft furnishings and cuddly toys. So has your child changed to a different type of

bedding recently? Are there lots of cuddly toys on the bed? Have any other allergens recently been introduced into the house, eg a new kitten or puppy or other furry animal?

- **Season**
  Many people's eczema is worse in cold weather.

- **Clothing**
  Eczema can flare up after wearing woollen clothing, both because wool is scratchy and because it may contain natural lanolin.

My child has severe eczema. I am very keen to try to find out if she is allergic to anything which might be making it worse. Can she be skin prick tested?

Skin prick testing might be helpful, as you may discover that your daughter is allergic to things which she could relatively easily avoid (allergen avoidance is discussed in Chapter 9). In particular, if your daughter is allergic to the house dust mite, decreasing the levels of this allergen in her bedroom may lead to a marked improvement in her eczema. We spend between one-third and one-half of our lives in bed, and old mattresses, pillows and duvets can contain extremely high levels of the house dust mite. Special bedding which prevents these mites coming into contact with the skin (discussed in more detail in the section on *House dust mite* in Chapter 9) can lead to a dramatic improvement in eczema. However, this bedding is quite expensive, and I would only recommend its use in people who are definitely allergic to house dust mite AND whose symptoms are difficult to control.

It is perfectly safe for your daughter to be skin prick tested, providing that she has a large enough eczema-free area of skin to be used for the testing. You will need to arrange it through your GP. Skin prick testing is quick (it takes about 15 minutes) and painless, but should always be done by someone who is expert in the procedure as it takes experience to interpret the results correctly. You will find more information about it in Appendix 1.

When my son's asthma is bad, his eczema is often much

better, and when his eczema is bad, his asthma is OK. Why is this?

Some people seem to have this seesaw experience with their asthma and eczema, although other people find that both conditions get worse together. Everyone with asthma and eczema has his or her own pattern which, incidentally, doesn't necessarily stay the same – so your son's pattern of symptoms may change as he grows older. At present, no one understands why any of this should happen, so the only consolation I can offer you is that at least for the time being you know what to expect.

Treatment for eczema

I thought the most effective treatment for eczema was steroid creams. I was very surprised when my doctor gave me a bath oil and an emollient to use on my daughter's skin, neither of which has got any steroid in it. Why is this?

Most children with eczema have dry skin, and in general dry skin tends to be less strong and more itchy than normal skin. If your daughter's skin is fragile, and she scratches it because it is itchy, then she will easily damage it and her eczema will become a great deal worse.

The bath oil and the emollient (moisturising and softening cream) your doctor has given you are intended to stop your daughter's skin being so dry. If her skin is not dry, it will be less itchy, and she will be less likely to scratch. If she does scratch, her skin will be less fragile and so less liable to damage.

The emollient should be used liberally all over your daughter's face and body at least twice a day, or as often as necessary. If her skin feels particularly itchy, suggest that she rubs in some emollient rather than scratching. The oil is intended for use in the bath but be careful – it can make the bath slippery. If possible, your daughter should avoid bubble baths and soap, as these both dry the skin and can also be irritating.

Steroid creams have their place in the treatment of eczema

(discussed later in this section), but their use should be kept down to the minimum possible.

My mother says that somebody with eczema should not have baths and should not go swimming. My GP says I should bath my son at least once a day using a bath oil. Who is right?

In some ways both your mother and your GP are right. Bathing with soap or with bubble bath can make eczema worse because these products dry the skin. However, if you use a dispersible bath oil in the water, and use either no soap at all or else a soap substitute such as emulsifying ointment, then bathing can be a convenient way of treating the skin. In addition, applying emollient creams straight after a bath when the skin is warm and soft is much more effective.

Your mother is right in saying that swimming can be bad for people with eczema. The problem is not the swimming, but the water in the pool! A number of chemicals such as chlorine are added to the water in swimming pools in order to disinfect it. However, if you are lucky enough to have access to a private swimming pool, there will probably be a much lower concentration of chemicals in the water and swimming there would be less likely to affect your son's skin. Swimming in the sea should also cause fewer problems than swimming in a pool (the salt water can be soothing), providing that you can find a clean beach where the water is not polluted.

Whenever I use a bath oil in the bath, my daughter, who has eczema, complains that the water stings her. Why is this happening?

Using a bath oil is an easy way to ensure that your daughter's skin remains well moisturised. However, certain of the bath oils made for use in eczema contain a high percentage of alcohol, and even when diluted in water this can sting. Don't stop using a bath oil, but ask your GP to change your daughter's prescription to one which does not contain alcohol.

My pharmacist tells me that the product I use for my

eczema comes as both an ointment and a cream. What is the difference, and which is best?

Ointments tend to be greasier than creams, and some people find these easier to apply accurately and sparingly. Others dislike the greasiness of an ointment and prefer a cream which tends to be absorbed by the skin more quickly. Which you use is a matter of personal preference, and may depend on whether you are using an emollient or a steroid preparation or both (emollients and steroid preparations are both discussed elsewhere in this section). For example, you might find that you prefer to use an ointment for your steroid preparation but a cream for your emollient.

When is the best time of day to use the skin cream my doctor has prescribed for my eczema?

This rather depends on how often you use your cream, and whether you are using an emollient or a steroid cream or both (emollients and steroid preparations are both discussed elsewhere in this section). In general, emollients (moisturising and softening creams) should be used twice a day every day whether your skin is bad or not, and most steroid creams are to be used two to three times a day when your skin needs them. Bath oils and soap substitutes should be used in the bath or the shower. You will find that emollients are better absorbed by your skin when it is warm, for example when you have just got out of a bath or shower. It is usually preferable to use your steroid cream after you have softened your skin with your emollient.

If your skin ever feels particularly itchy, a good remedy is to gently rub in a generous amount of your emollient. This is very much better than scratching.

I have heard a lot of worrying things about steroids. I'm concerned about this as my doctor has given me a steroid cream for my eczema. Are steroid creams safe to use on the skin?

Nearly all medications have side effects, even the ones we take for granted such as aspirin and paracetamol. Steroid medications are no exception to this so, as a general rule, they should be used as sparingly as possible. Your doctor will only have prescribed a steroid cream for you if it is really needed, and then only in the minimum strength and amount necessary to bring about an improvement in your skin. If you use your steroid cream as directed by your doctor – only using it on the worst areas of your skin and only for as long as it takes to clear your eczema – then there should be no harmful effects. Some of the milder creams are now available for you to buy over the counter at your chemist, which indicates that they are safe enough for occasional use without a doctor's supervision.

The possible side effects of steroid creams are most commonly seen on the skin itself. If they are used for a long time or in large amounts, the skin can become reddened and thin, and marks like stretch marks can appear. Facial skin is the most vulnerable to these effects, so you should take care to use only the mildest steroid creams (ie 0.5% hydrocortisone) on your face, and if this doesn't clear things up, you should see your doctor. The skin can also become pale, or may seem more hairy. If the creams are used in very large amounts, there may be an effect on the body's production of its own natural steroid hormones, leading to a deficiency of these hormones which can reduce growth in children, although this is VERY rare.

There are now new steroid creams available which have fewer serious side effects because they are not absorbed by the skin as much as the older types. Two examples are mometasone furoate (brand name Elocon) and fluticasone propionate (brand name Cutivate). If you use only small amounts of steroid cream, then there is no need for you to change from your usual brand, as you are at so little risk from side effects. The need for a change will only arise if you are using large amounts of steroids, either because you have very bad eczema and use a lot of your cream, or because you have asthma or hayfever as well and also use steroid treatments for those. If this is the case, your GP might want to consider changing your prescription to one of these new creams, and you could discuss this when you next visit the doctor's. Obviously no one should alter their own treatment without first discussing it with their doctor: waiting a couple of days for an appointment cannot cause any harm.

Incidentally, the steroids that are used in treating eczema are not the same as those abused by some athletes – those are anabolic steroids, while the ones used for eczema are a different type called corticosteroids. Confusion can arise because both are referred to by the abbreviation 'steroids'.

My eczema is much better when I take prednisolone tablets for my asthma. Why can't I take these all of the time?

Prednisolone is a corticosteroid which is taken in tablet form for acute attacks of asthma. Like you, most people find it very effective in these circumstances, but if you take it over a long period of time (which means months or years) it can cause unwanted side effects. These include weight gain, thinning of the skin, thinning of the bones (osteoporosis) and other serious problems. None of these problems is common, but all are recognised long-term risks of taking oral steroids. Doctors therefore prescribe these drugs to be taken for as short a period as possible, which usually means for less than two weeks at a time and ideally not more than four times a year: they are then safe and effective treatments, which can even be life-saving in acute asthma.

Your eczema will almost always get better when you are taking an oral steroid medication such as prednisolone because the drug is carried by your blood stream to every part of your body, including your skin. However, the possible side effects mean that oral steroids should not be prescribed for eczema, as it would be rather like using a sledgehammer to crack a nut! Instead, you should concentrate on avoiding the factors that make your eczema worse, and use plenty of emollient (moisturising and softening cream) regularly to make your skin stronger and more flexible, using steroid creams only on the worst affected areas. This way you will get the best improvement with the minimum side effects.

Just when my son's eczema seems to be under control he starts scratching and we are back to square one. What can I do?

You may find the following suggestions helpful.

- Try to make sure that your son is not coming into contact with trigger factors which could be making his eczema worse. It might be that there are certain things that you only allow him to do when his skin is particularly good, such as swimming in a chlorinated pool or horse riding, and it could be these that are undoing all of your good work.
- Make sure that you continue to use emollient (moisturising and softening) creams even when your son's skin is trouble-free. Keeping his skin well moisturised will help to protect it from damage.
- Ensure that your son can't damage his skin so much when he scratches. Make sure that his fingernails are kept short and smooth, and that he does not wear irritant clothing such as wool or other scratchy fabrics.
- If necessary, you can help to reduce the itching by the use of antihistamine preparations. It is best to ask your doctor to prescribe these for your son, as many of the antihistamines which can be bought from a chemist can cause drowsiness, whereas the newer types (most of which are only available on prescription) do not have this sedating effect.
- Avoid using calamine lotion. Although it is a traditional remedy for itchy skin, it is messy and not very effective.

My daughter has very severe eczema. Despite using the skin cream, the bath oil and the steroid cream prescribed by my doctor, it is not getting any better. What else can I do?

Firstly, it is important to check that you are using your daughter's skin treatments correctly. If you are in any doubt about this, check with your doctor. Assuming that you are, it might be that there is something in one of these creams which affects your daughter's skin, and this could be making her skin worse instead of better. If you think that any of the following applies to your daughter's eczema medication, then talk to your GP about altering her prescription.

- Some emollients (moisturising and softening creams) contain lanolin or parabens, and these are chemicals which can irritate some people's skin. It would be sensible to change to an emollient which is lanolin and parabens free.

- If your daughter has very inflamed and broken skin, the bath oil might actually be causing irritation, as some of them contain a high concentration of alcohol. You should consider changing to a bath oil which has less alcohol in it, or one which is alcohol-free.
- Steroid creams are available in various strengths, and it may be that the one prescribed for your daughter is relatively weak. Sometimes changing temporarily to a stronger steroid cream will solve the problem.

There might be other avoidable triggers which are making your daughter's eczema worse. The following list is not comprehensive, but it may help you to track down the specific cause.

- If your daughter is particularly allergic to the house dust mite and is regularly being exposed to this allergen, her eczema will not have the chance to get better. Some people find that their eczema improves when they take measures to avoid the house dust mite, either by reducing overall mite levels, or by using mattress, duvet and pillow covers aimed at reducing contact between the house dust mite and the skin. You will find more information about dealing with house dust mites in Chapter 9.
- Similarly, the allergens from animals such as dogs, cats and rabbits can make eczema worse, and it would be sensible to make sure your daughter does not have contact with these animal allergens.
- She may be coming into contact with certain chemicals which make her skin worse, for example the chlorine in swimming pools, the fragrances in toiletries (eg soaps and shampoos) and the additives in washing powders. You might consider changing your washing powder to one which is as free as possible from additives such as enzymes.
- Her skin will almost certainly feel more comfortable if she wears natural fibres, particularly cotton. However, woollen clothing may be a problem, both because wool is scratchy and because it may contain natural lanolin.

Some people with severe eczema occasionally get a mild but persistent skin infection. If this is the case, the eczema will not clear properly until the infection is treated. This is best done by a relatively long (several weeks) course of a particular oral antibiotic, which your doctor could prescribe.

Remember that stress is a factor which often makes eczema worse. It might be worth looking into whether or not your daughter is happy at school by having a word with her teachers.

My son's eczema has been really bad recently and our GP has prescribed antibiotics. Why?

When the skin becomes damaged and inflamed, it is much more vulnerable to becoming infected by the germs which live on our skin and which usually cause no harm. The infection is usually mild, and can easily be confused with the inflammation caused by the eczema itself. The commonest germ causing this type of infection is called *Staphylococcus*, and this responds well to treatment with a suitable antibiotic. Your son's eczema is much more likely to clear up once the infection has been treated.

I have heard that evening primrose oil might improve my eczema. Is this true?

Recent research has shown us that people with eczema may not have an adequate natural supply of certain chemicals which prevent inflammation and which are usually found in the body. As a plentiful supply of these chemicals can be found in evening primrose oil, further research has been carried out to see if taking this oil can help people with eczema. The results have been somewhat inconclusive: the oil has to be taken in large amounts, and does not seem to be effective in everyone. However, you may think that it is worth trying it to see if it helps you.

My eczema, which is pretty bad, usually gets better when I go on holiday (I like to go to warm, sunny places). Because of this, my skin specialist has suggested that I try a

treatment called PUVA. I didn't really understand his explanation of this. What is it, and will it work?

PUVA stands for 'psoralen plus ultra-violet A'. If this is how it was described to you I'm not surprised that you didn't understand! PUVA is a treatment in which a plant extract called psoralen is taken by mouth. Two hours later you are asked to lie or sit under a machine rather like a sun lamp, which produces a certain type of light called ultra-violet A. This treatment can be very useful in a number of skin conditions, including eczema and psoriasis, and it may produce a big improvement. However, if it is used over a long period of time it carries all the same risks as overexposure to the sun's rays, for example ageing of the skin and skin cancers. Because of this, doctors recommend that it is only used to get eczema under control and not as a long-term treatment.

Diet and eczema

Can certain foods make my eczema worse?

Approximately 25% of people with severe eczema have a true food allergy to such foods as eggs, milk, wheat, nuts and fish. As well as the symptoms associated with food allergy (such as swelling of the mouth and face, generalised itchiness, wheezing and bowel problems), these people may also describe symptoms occurring as much as 48 hours later, such as continued itching and worsening of eczema.

In children under 5 years old, eating foods containing cow's milk and hen's eggs may make the symptoms of eczema worse. It is unlikely that these foodstuffs are the sole cause of their eczema, but for these children, eliminating the food responsible from the diet may cause a dramatic improvement in their condition. In adults, food allergy is not usually the only cause of eczema, and it is unlikely that avoiding particular foods will cure your problems.

Food allergy is discussed in more detail in Chapter 5.

Are there any foodstuffs which should be avoided in the diet of a child with eczema?

Some foods are more likely than others to cause allergies, and these include cow's milk and eggs. However, I would not recommend that you automatically exclude these from your child's diet. They are both good sources of protein, and milk is an important source of calcium, which is essential for bone growth in children. Few milk substitutes contains as much calcium as cow's milk. In addition, relatively few children respond to these restricted diets, which can be both expensive and difficult to follow (it is not always easy to know which foodstuffs contain eggs and cow's milk).

A more logical approach would be to find out whether your child is allergic to any foodstuffs and then to avoid those. However, this can be difficult, as small children do not always show their allergies on skin prick testing (you will find more information about these tests in Appendix 1). It may even be impossible to identify problem foods because there is often a 48-hour gap between the food being eaten and eczema worsening.

I would suggest that you decide, with the help of your doctor, whether your child's eczema is being adequately controlled by the use of skin creams and bath oils. If not, your doctor will be guided by the results of skin prick tests and RAST (also explained in Appendix 1) whether it is worthwhile considering an exclusion diet, as explained in the section on *Food allergens* in Chapter 9. You will find the advice of a dietician very helpful if you decide to go along this route.

My 1-year-old daughter has eczema, and my health visitor has told me to start her on a cow's milk free diet. I am not particularly keen on this, as I feel that milk is an important part of her diet. Can a cow's milk free diet help, and is it safe?

You are right, milk is an important part of a young child's diet. I would suggest that before you embark on a cow's milk free diet (which can be quite difficult to keep to), you find out whether or not your daughter is truly allergic to cow's milk.

If I were to see your child, I would ask you for the history of her problems, I would examine her, and I would then suggest skin prick testing her to various food products. I might also send off a blood sample for a RAST to cow's milk, which is a specific test for this allergy. All these tests are explained fully in Appendix 1.

I would only suggest a cow's milk free diet if we found good evidence that your child was allergic to it. If this were the case, I would suggest that you consulted a dietician, both to learn which foodstuffs you would need to avoid (it is not always obvious which foods contain cow's milk) and to ensure that your daughter ate a diet which was adequate in calcium, protein and calories.

I have tried to help my child's eczema by excluding foods from his diet which I think might be making him worse, but his eczema is as bad as ever. He is now on a very limited diet but I am frightened of reintroducing all of these foods in case he gets even worse. What should I do?

This is quite a common problem. You have tried your best to improve your son's eczema, but unfortunately your methods did not work. As you have seen no real improvement after excluding all these foods, it is unlikely that you will make him worse by reintroducing them. And as you will see from the earlier sections in this chapter, it is likely that there are many other factors apart from foodstuffs which are responsible for your son's eczema.

I would suggest that you reintroduce the excluded foods one at a time, starting with the most nutritionally important foods such as cow's milk and other forms of protein (although I would suggest that for the time being you avoid egg). If you add one new food to your son's diet every three days it will give you sufficient time to identify a problem should one occur. I would also suggest that you consult your GP, as there may be other ways to help your son's eczema that you haven't yet considered.

I am sure that there are certain things that I eat that make my eczema worse but I can't seem to be able to work out which. What can I do?

If you suspect only a small number of foods of causing your

problems, you might consider eliminating all of them from your diet for a trial period of approximately two weeks, to see whether or not there is an improvement. If your eczema does improve, you could then reintroduce them one at a time, with an interval of at least three days between each food, and this way you should be able to spot which one is causing your problems. You will need to remember that there will be a timelag of approximately 48 hours between eating a foodstuff and the flare up of your symptoms. You should also bear in mind that there are a large number of other things that can affect your eczema, and that a flare up could be due to one of these as opposed to one of the foods which you are testing. Please be careful not to exclude too many items from your diet at a time, and to ensure that you are at all times eating a nutritionally balanced diet.

An alternative approach would be to consult your GP and to ask if he would consider arranging for you to have diagnostic testing such as RAST or skin prick testing (both explained in detail in Appendix 1). The foods most commonly associated with true allergy are all proteins such as peanut, egg and milk, and so it is likely that you would be tested for these foodstuffs first.

If you don't yet have any idea which foodstuffs might be responsible, then I suggest that you start to keep a food diary of everything you eat and how bad your eczema is, to see if there is any relationship between them. This will be easier to do if you do not eat pre-prepared and convenience foods (which contain large numbers of ingredients, not all of which are easy to identify) but stick instead to fresh produce and home cooking. Again there may be an interval of up to 48 hours between eating a food and seeing a reaction. Take this diary with you when you see your doctor, as it will help you both to decide which foods you might need to try eliminating from your diet or which might be worth considering for diagnostic testing.

Living with eczema

My child, who has eczema, has developed pale areas of skin on her face and behind her knees. What causes this?

Eczema itself can cause depigmentation (loss of the natural colour of the skin) but another cause of this is the use of steroid creams. This depigmentation is particularly noticeable when an area of eczema has just recently cleared, but it should become less marked with time. Make sure that you use as little steroid cream as is needed to keep the eczema under control. You will find more information about the use of these creams in the section on *Treatment for eczema* earlier in this chapter.

I had eczema as a child. Now I only get problems with my skin when I'm abroad on holiday. Do you have any ideas why this might be?

There are several things which might be troubling your skin whilst you are away on holiday. If you go somewhere warm and sunny, it might be sunlight which is causing your problems.

- Polymorphic light eruption is a reaction of the skin to sunlight which takes the form of an itchy red rash or blisters which occur particularly on the face, chest, hands, arms and legs. To avoid this, you should keep out of the sun as much as possible, and you must use a high factor sunscreen when you are in the sun.
- In some people, exposure to sunlight (especially when the weather is humid) can cause 'prickly heat', in which the skin becomes inflamed and the sweat produced by the sweat glands becomes trapped under the skin's surface. This can be quite a problem for someone with delicate or sensitive skin.
- Urticaria (discussed in the section on *Skin allergies explained* at the beginning of this chapter) can also be triggered by sunlight in some people. A diffuse red rash and itchy weals oocur, particularly in areas which are only rarely exposed to the sun. The reaction is rapid, developing within minutes, occurs only on parts of the body which have been exposed, and disappears within an hour.

Other things apart from the sun might be causing your problem. The following list may help you to discover what they are.

- You might be using certain creams on your skin which you do not use during the rest of the year, for example a sunblock, sunscreen or an after-sun preparation. These could contain chemicals which affect your skin.
- Your diet is likely to be different when you are on holiday, and it could be that you are eating more of certain foods (such as shellfish or cheese) which could be affecting your skin.
- You could be coming into contact with substances to which you are allergic but which you don't usually meet at home. Examples include certain plants and flowers, or a different type of washing powder or starch used on the hotel's sheets.

If you can track down which of these things is causing your problem, most of them are quite easy to avoid. Failing this, make sure that you take appropriate treatment for your eczema on holiday with you.

Why does my son's eczema always get better when we go abroad on holiday?

This could be happening because he is no longer in contact with whatever it is at home that makes his eczema worse, or because he is encountering something on holiday which makes it better – or it could be a combination of the two! Earlier sections in this chapter have described the factors which can make eczema worse, including allergens, foods, skin preparations and certain chemicals. The change of environment during your holiday may mean that your son's exposure to one or more of these triggers is reduced. It might simply be that he feels less stressed when he is on holiday. Alternatively, it might be the change in the climate which is helpful: increased humidity and increased amounts of sunlight can both help people with eczema.

Is it true that exposure to the house dust mite can make my eczema worse? If so, how can I avoid it?

It does seem that there are specific allergens which can make eczema worse, and the house dust mite is definitely a culprit. Approximately 75% of people with severe eczema are allergic to this allergen and, if you are one of them, your eczema may be dramatically improved by house dust mite avoidance measures. In particular, decreasing the levels of house dust mite in your mattress and bedding can lead to a significant improvement. This is because when you are in bed, your skin is in close contact with very high levels of the allergen, which can be particularly troublesome if your skin is inflamed or broken.

The reasons why the house dust mite is such a problem for people with allergies is explained in the section on *Triggers* in Chapter 1, and ways to reduce your contact with it are discussed in Chapter 9.

I have heard that it is dangerous for a child with eczema to be exposed to the cold sore virus. Is this true?

If you have eczema, your skin is more vulnerable to all types of infection, including infection with bacteria or viruses. If children with severe eczema catch the cold sore virus or the chickenpox virus, they can be particularly badly affected so, wherever possible, contact with these viruses should be avoided.

A medication which can combat these two viruses now exists. It is called acyclovir (brand name Zovirax) and is very effective in overcoming this problem. If your child has severe eczema and develops chickenpox or any other rash with water-filled blisters, take him or her straight to your doctor as a course of this antivirus drug may make a big difference.

We have a cat. Could this be making my daughter's eczema worse?

Yes, it could. Cats produce a very potent allergen in their saliva, which they then spread over their bodies as they groom themselves with their tongues. Both direct contact with the cat (by stroking it) and indirect contact (through shed hair and skin particles) are likely to make your child's eczema worse. It only takes a very small amount of the allergen to do this, so the cat could be responsible even if he lives outside most of the time.

It is unlikely that the cat is the only trigger factor for your daughter's eczema, and only you can decide whether or not to keep the pet at home. It might be helpful to ask yourself whether or not your child's eczema gets better when she and the cat are not in contact, for example when you are on holiday. Rather than get rid of the cat, you might prefer to find a temporary alternative home for him and then see if there is any change in your daughter's eczema. However, you will need to remember that it may take many months of thorough cleaning to remove all traces of the cat allergen from your home.

Dermatitis

My doctor has told me that the skin rash on my hands is contact dermatitis. What could be causing this?

If your rash is only on your hands, it is quite likely that it is due to allergic contact dermatitis, and not to eczema (the difference between these conditions was discussed in the section on *Skin allergies explained* at the beginning of this chapter). The appearance of skin affected by dermatitis can resemble that affected by eczema, in that it may be red, inflamed and sore, with open areas or scabs. However, in allergic contact dermatitis, the skin rash only appears on the area of skin which has been in contact with the substance which caused the reaction. It usually appears 1-3 days after contact with the allergen responsible.

Common allergens known to cause dermatitis include:

- fragrances in soaps and toiletries;
- chemicals such as lanolin and parabens found in creams and ointments;
- metals such as nickel and cobalt found in jewellery, zip fasteners, jean studs and so on;
- chromate in tanned leather, matches and green clothes dyes;
- formaldehyde found in cosmetics, newsprint, fabric softeners and cigarettes;
- plants such as primula obconica (a member of the primrose family), chrysanthemums, ivy and tulip bulbs; and
- rubber products, especially boots and gloves, which contain mecaptobenzothiazole and thiurams.

It may now be obvious to you what is causing your allergic

contact dermatitis. If not, you could ask your GP to refer you to a dermatologist, as patch testing (explained in detail in Appendix 1) may be useful.

I believe that my dermatitis is caused by a chemical I use in my work as a hairdresser. How can I prove this?

Hairdressers come into contact with a number of chemicals during their work, so it is quite possible that your dermatitis is being caused by one or more of them. If this is the case, then your hands should improve a great deal when you are on holiday and away from work, or when you wear plastic gloves to handle the chemicals. Avoid latex gloves as these themselves can cause an allergic reaction.

As to identifying which chemical is the culprit, the only sure way of finding out is by patch testing (explained in detail in Appendix 1), which your doctor can organise for you. Special sets of allergens are available for testing people who work in occupations such as hairdressing.

Once the substances causing your dermatitis have been identified, it is important that you are told where they are commonly found, and how to avoid them. If you are allergic to one of the chemicals at work, then you will need to talk to you employer about how you can avoid coming into contact with it.

I have suddenly developed dermatitis. The only possible cause I can think of is a skin cream, but I have been using this for months with no problem. Is this possible?

One of the puzzling things about allergic contact dermatitis is that a reaction can occur to a substance which you have previously used for a long time without any problems. Why an allergy can suddenly develop like this is something we do not yet understand.

It is perfectly possible that you have developed a reaction to your skin cream despite having used it happily for several months. I suggest you stop using it and see if your dermatitis gets better. If it doesn't, then another substance is at fault, and you may need the help of a dermatologist (skin specialist) to discover what it is.

What are hypoallergenic cosmetic products? Why are they so expensive?

Every time you put a product containing chemicals in contact with your skin, you are effectively challenging your skin to react to it. If you are prone to allergies, then you risk developing a reaction to any of the substances contained in the product. Most toiletries and cosmetics contain a wide range of ingredients which can act as allergens. 'Hypo' simply means 'less than' or 'lower in', so hypoallergenic products are lower in allergens than the conventional formulations. They are free from the commonest substances known to cause allergic reactions, such as perfumes, colourings and preservatives. This does not mean that they are completely allergen-free, but they are more likely to be well tolerated by people with allergies.

They can cost more than the equivalent conventional products both because they are made in smaller quantities and because the manufacturer may have to use more expensive ingredients. However, several chain stores are beginning to market their own brands of hypoallergenic products which are more competitively priced, and it would be worth you looking out for these.

Beware 'fragrance-free' products: these are allowed to contain a number of chemicals which mask the smell of the other ingredients. Instead use products described as 'unperfumed', as these have no perfumes or fragrances added.

I am a vegetarian. Are there any hypoallergenic cosmetics which have not been tested on animals?

Various ranges of skin care, make-up and other cosmetic products are now available which claim to be 'animal-compassionate' or 'against animal testing'. Only you can decide whether any of these ranges meet your ethical criteria, based on the information given in their leaflets and other publicity material.

Very few of these products are also labelled as hypoallergenic. However, most of the companies which produce them have always been very good at listing all the ingredients used on the labels on their packaging, and some invite customers to write to them with any queries about their products. If you know which substances cause you problems with your dermatitis, then you may be able to use this information to help you choose suitable cosmetics which will not aggravate your skin.

I can't always find the make-up I want in hypoallergenic ranges, so what do you suggest I do?

A recent change in the law will perhaps help to give you a wider choice of make-up, as manufacturers are now legally required to list every ingredient of these products. I suggest you read the labels very carefully, and so avoid any cosmetics which contain substances which you know trigger your allergy.

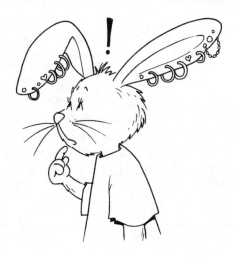

I have pierced ears, and I've noticed that some of my earrings make them very sore and itchy while others don't. Why?

I suspect that the fastenings of some of your earrings are made from nickel, that you are allergic to it, and that you therefore have a form of allergic contact dermatitis called nickel dermatitis. The earrings which do not affect you are probably made of gold, silver or stainless steel.

Nickel is commonly found in earrings and other jewellery; in clothing fasteners such as buckles, hooks and eyes, zips and jean studs; and also in spectacle frames, coins and some household utensils. In this country as many as one in every 10 women are allergic to it, and when they come into contact with products containing nickel, they develop inflamed skin within 1-3 days. This reaction is localised to the area in contact with the nickel, but it can be very angry and sore.

I suggest that when you buy earrings in future you check very carefully to see what they are made from, and only buy them if you are sure that they do not contain nickel. It is interesting to note that because of this problem of contact dermatitis, in Scandinavia it is illegal to sell earrings or other items of jewellery which contain nickel.

Testing has shown me to be allergic to formaldehyde. I have never even heard of this. What is it, and what substances contain formaldehyde?

Formaldehyde is a chemical which is found in many everyday items such as fabric softeners, newspapers, cigarettes, crease-resistant clothing, cosmetics and some preservatives. If your allergy is severe, you may need the help and advice of a dermatologist (skin specialist), and your doctor can arrange a referral.

Please can you tell me what is in sticking plasters which causes me to come out in a red rash?

This could be due to a number of things. Sticking plasters can contain zinc, antiseptics and fragrances, and all use adhesives. Any of these can cause an allergic reaction. Hypoallergenic sticking plasters are now widely available, but if you are affected even by these, you could try using dry gauze and a hypoallergenic adhesive paper tape instead.

I'm a keen gardener, but I also get dermatitis. How can I best look after my skin?

First, be careful in your choice of plants. As a number of plants can cause contact dermatitis (particularly chrysanthemums and various other members of the daisy family), as from 1995 all such plants on sale will have been clearly labelled with the information that they can cause skin irritation. This information may be in very small print on the label or seed packet!

Second, always wear gloves when you are gardening, avoid rubbing your eyes and face, and don't use a strimmer, which can throw sap and fibres into your face.

I have worked as a nurse for many years, but recently seemed to have developed an allergic reaction to rubber gloves. Is it possible to develop an allergy after using the same type of gloves for years? And what treatment is available for my problem?

Yes, it is possible to develop an allergy to something you have previously used over many years without any problems. We do not know why it is that the body can suddenly develop such an allergy, but once this has happened, the only effective treatment involves avoiding the substance concerned. You are most likely to be allergic to a chemical such as mecaptobenzothiazole or a thiuram that is actually in the rubber itself. However, it could be something else in the gloves that is causing your allergy, such as the starch powder used to make them easier to put on. Almost 5% of all hospital workers have been found to be allergic to latex, which can cause both eczema and asthma as well as dermatitis.

In the first instance you could try changing to a different brand of glove. In particular there are certain brands of plastic glove which are made specifically for people with sensitive skins or allergies to rubber products. In addition you should treat the affected areas with an appropriate steroid cream. However, the only really effective treatment is to avoid the source of your problem, and it might be that you have to avoid tasks that require the use of protective gloves.

4
Hayfever

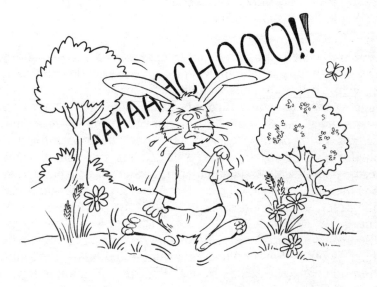

Introduction

The term hayfever was originally used to describe the symptoms suffered by farm workers during haymaking, but what we now regard as hayfever has nothing to do with either hay or having a fever. It is a very misleading name: fever is rare, and the causes include a large number of allergens other than hay.

Hayfever is very common, and is thought to affect up to a quarter of the population at some time during each year.

Although it is not life-threatening, it causes a great deal of misery. I hope it will be useful for you to learn more about your hayfever, as this should make it possible for you to work out which allergens are causing your problems, to reduce your exposure to the culprits, and discover how best to manage any remaining symptoms you may have.

Hayfever explained

What exactly is hayfever?

If you have hayfever, you are allergic to one of the aero-allergens (allergens with particles light enough to be carried through the air). When this allergen is present in the air you are breathing, the lining of your nose and throat become inflamed (the process of inflammation is explained in the section on *Symptoms* in Chapter 1). In many people, hayfever is due to an allergy to a specific type of plant pollen. This causes a seasonal problem, more correctly called seasonal allergic rhinitis. The name rhinitis comes from the Greek: 'rhinos' means 'nose' and '-itis' means 'inflammation', so rhinitis is inflammation of the lining of the nose.

Sometimes hayfever symptoms can be caused by an allergy to allergens other than pollens, for example the house dust mite or animal dander (the scales from their hair or fur, something like dandruff in humans). These allergens are not seasonal but occur all year round, causing continual symptoms throughout the four seasons. The correct medical term for this problem is perennial allergic rhinitis. It is, of course, possible for you to be allergic to more than one allergen, and so your symptoms may vary throughout the year.

There is more information about the allergens which can cause hayfever in the section on *Triggers* later in this chapter.

How do pollens cause hayfever?

Once you have become allergic to a particular pollen, an allergic reaction is triggered the next time that those pollen grains come

into contact with the lining of your nose and throat or the
membranes covering your eyes. The pollen grains contain a
substance which stimulates the cells of your immune system,
which release histamine and other chemicals, causing the small
blood vessels in the affected parts of your body to enlarge. Fluid
leaking from these enlarged blood vessels causes swelling and
irritation, leading to the typical hayfever symptoms of a runny or
stuffed-up nose, sneezing and watery eyes.

You specifically asked about pollens, but the same reaction
would occur if you had the all-year-round type of hayfever (as
explained in the answer to the previous question): only the
allergen causing your symptoms would be different. The allergic
process involved is the same as that discussed in more detail in
the section on *Allergy explained* in Chapter 1, where you will
also find more information on histamine and the immune system.

**My daughter, who has asthma, is now 9 years old, and has
no sign of hayfever. Does this mean that she has escaped it?**

Hayfever can start at any time of life, although it is most common
between the ages of 8 and 25 years. I am afraid it is therefore still
possible that your daughter might develop it. If she does so, it is
important that it is treated, as hayfever can make asthma worse.

Is hayfever getting more common?

Yes, just as with the other allergic disorders, there seems to be an
increase in the number of people with hayfever. Increased levels
of air pollution may be partly to blame, as damage to the
membranes of the eye and nose by these pollutants might make
the allergic effect of pollens more potent.

Is it really hayfever?

Is a runny, itchy nose always due to hayfever?

No, there are a number of other problems which can mimic
hayfever. These include:

• the common cold;

- vasomotor rhinitis, a problem of the small blood vessels supplying the nose which is nothing to do with allergy;
- nasal polyps, which are small harmless outgrowths of the lining of the nose which can cause a blocked or runny nose; and
- rhinitis medicamentosa, a problem caused by the overuse of nasal decongestants.

How can I tell whether I have a cold or whether my hayfever is playing up?

Sometimes this can be very difficult. Usually, however, a cold goes through definite stages. It starts with a feeling of itchiness in the nose and throat, and a general feeling of being poorly; it then moves onto a stage of having a very runny nose; and it finishes with a couple of days when the secretions from the nose become thick and discoloured, and the nose itself rather crusty. A cold generally lasts 3-6 days, and then disappears.

In hayfever, the nasal secretions are usually thin and clear and watery, and the symptoms do not pass through these clear-cut stages. However, in severe hayfever, the nasal secretions can be yellow or even green in colour, and you may feel quite unwell, making it hard to tell the difference.

During the hayfever season, for me June and July, I often get the feeling of having a tight chest, which gets worse with exercise. I had always thought that this was part and parcel of my hayfever, but now my GP has diagnosed asthma. Is this right?

If you think about it, you will realise that the lining of your nose and throat meets up with the lining of your windpipe and lungs. They form one continuous system. If there is an allergic process going on in the lining of your nose, it is not surprising that the lining of your lungs could be affected by the same allergen. Inflammation in the lungs causes the symptoms of asthma, hence your feeling of chest tightness (a common symptom of mild asthma).

So the answer to your question is yes, I think your GP is right in diagnosing asthma. It would be worthwhile asking him

whether he thinks you might benefit from treatment specifically
for this, which, if your symptoms are seasonal, could be taken at
the relevant times of year rather than all year round. Effective
treatment of your hayfever itself will also reduce the symptoms
you get from your chest.

Symptoms

What are the symptoms of hayfever?

Common symptoms of hayfever are:

* sneezing;
* a runny or stuffy nose;
* itching of the eyes, nose and throat;
* watery, inflamed eyes (conjunctivitis);
* a dark appearance under the eyes (allergic shiners) due to
  inflammation in the sinuses; and
* loss of sense of smell.

If you have hayfever, these symptoms often combine to make you
feel tired, lethargic and generally under the weather. You may
find it is difficult to sleep well, and your enjoyment of many
aspects of life including eating, sporting activities and anything to
do with the outdoors can be affected. You may find that your
concentration is impaired, and your performance at school or at
work can be affected.

**I have never had hayfever, so I find it difficult to
understand why my husband gets so irritable when his
hayfever is at its worst. What does having hayfever feel
like?**

The symptoms of hayfever range from a few sneezes right
through to a condition which affects the whole body. In severe
cases, people with hayfever feel as if they have a bad head cold
with a fever, although their body temperature is normal. It sounds
as if your husband has fairly bad hayfever.

Imagine a head cold at its worst phase, when your eyes and

nose feel intensely irritated and itchy, and your head as if it is about to explode. Your nose runs constantly, but at the same time feels stuffy and blocked up. Your nose quickly becomes red and sore, and the constant sneezing is embarrassing. Your sinuses may be blocked, leading to quite severe pain in your face and loss of your sense of smell. On top of all of this you would probably be feeling tired and irritable, which could lead to a degree of depression. This is probably how your husband feels, so it is no wonder he is not at his best during his hayfever season.

For me, one of the worst things about my hayfever is the way that my nose runs. Some days it is so bad it is quite embarrassing. Why does this happen?

When the lining of your nose is irritated by pollen grains or other allergens to which it is allergic, it becomes inflamed (tissue inflammation is discussed in more detail in the section on *Symptoms* in Chapter 1). This inflammation causes swelling in the lining of your nose and leakiness of the small blood vessels there. Your nose also produces more mucus. The combination of the leaking fluid and the mucus can make your nose feel stuffy, can make it run (as in your case), or can do both at the same time. Your GP should be able to prescribe some treatment for you which should considerably reduce your symptoms.

Why does my nose itch when my hayfever is bad?

The inflammation of the lining of the nose which results from contact with pollen in people who have hayfever comes from the release of certain chemicals in the body, including histamine (there is more about histamine in the section on *Allergy explained* in Chapter 1). One of the effects of histamine is itchiness. So, in the same way that an insect bite itches, the nose can itch. Histamine production in the nose can also lead to sneezing, and in hayfever this can occur in bouts of between five and 20 sneezes.

Some people also find that their ears itch. This is not due to histamine or to pollen landing in the ears, but is the result of irritation of a nerve which supplies both the back of the throat and the ear.

When my hayfever is at its worst, my nose feels completely blocked, but blowing my nose does not seem to make it any better. Why is this?

The blocked feeling in your nose is mainly due to swelling of the tissues rather than to blockage by mucous secretions. Because of this, no amount of blowing can relieve it. In fact, blowing your nose too much or too hard can actually make the problem worse.

A completely blocked nose not only causes local discomfort but can also lead to headaches, disturbed sleep, and a sore throat first thing in the morning (because of breathing through your mouth during the night). Because of this, I think that you should see your GP, who will be able to suggest some effective treatment for your hayfever which will help with this symptom.

Why do I sometimes get pain above my eyebrows and beneath my eyes during the hayfever season?

The bones of your face are not solid, but have hollow spaces in them called sinuses, which are joined to the air passages of the nose by small openings. Air usually passes freely from the nose into the sinuses. However, when the lining of the nose is inflamed (as during a cold or during an attack of hayfever) the openings of the sinuses can become blocked and their drainage system disturbed. Once blocked, the pressure in the sinuses can increase because of the accumulation of secretions. The increase in pressure within these bony cavities can then cause severe pain which can be felt above the eyebrows, either side of the nose, or in the upper teeth.

My son had a severe nosebleed one day when his hayfever was particularly bad. I found this very alarming, as there seemed to be a huge amount of blood and I did not know what to do. Why did this nosebleed happen and what should I do if one happens again?

One of the functions of the nose is to moisten and to warm the air as it is breathed in so that it does not irritate the lungs. To do this, the lining of the nose is well supplied with blood vessels, which provide both the heat and the moisture. In hayfever, the swelling of the lining of the nose can make it more fragile than normal, and it is more easily damaged. Even quite minor damage to the lining can rupture one of the blood vessels there, which leads to a nosebleed.

The blood loss in a nosebleed always appears to be greater than it really is, so try not to be too alarmed if it happens to your son again. This is what you should do.

- Keep calm.
- Squeeze your son's nose firmly both sides of the bony bridge and maintain firm pressure until the bleeding stops.
- Do not let him blow his nose, even if it feels uncomfortably blocked.
- Mop up any blood escaping from his nostrils gently with a handkerchief or paper tissue.
- If the bleeding does not settle within 10-15 minutes then consider seeking medical attention.

If these nosebleeds happen frequently, it would be wise to ask your GP to check your son, to rule out any causes other than his hayfever which might require attention, or to prescribe suitable treatment.

Why do I get a sore throat when I have hayfever?

Normally you breathe through your nose, which is designed to moisten and warm the air passing through it. During an episode of hayfever, your nose will generally be blocked, and you will therefore tend to breathe through your mouth. Your mouth is less efficient than your nose in moistening and warming the air, and so your throat can become irritated by the drier air passing through it.

The best way to avoid this is to take adequate treatment for your hayfever, although a short-term answer would be to gargle with a soluble aspirin or paracetamol solution, which will help relieve the soreness. However, parents should remember that aspirin and aspirin-containing preparations should not be used by children under 12 years old.

When my hayfever is at its worst, I have all the symptoms of a cold, including yellowy-green catarrh and a sore throat. When I asked my doctor for antibiotics he would not give them to me. Why is this?

The symptoms you have described could be due to either hayfever or a cold. Antibiotics are not helpful in hayfever unless the sinuses (the hollow spaces in the bones of the face) are infected. Even if your doctor thought that you had a cold, antibiotics would not be the right treatment. Colds are caused by an infection with a virus and viruses cannot, sadly, be treated using antibiotics. As all antibiotics can have side effects, including skin rashes, tummy upsets and diarrhoea, your doctor will try to prescribe them only when they are really necessary and likely to have a positive effect.

Why, if hayfever affects my nose, do I seem to produce thick catarrh from my chest?

Your nose, throat and windpipe are part of one continuous passage. Mucus and watery secretions produced in your nose can drip down the back of your throat and cause you to cough. It may feel as if you are coughing the catarrh up from your lungs, but it is most likely that actually it is being produced from your nose. This can be a very unpleasant feeling, and I would suggest that you consult your GP, who can prescribe treatments that will help to reduce this problem.

During the hayfever season I have noticed that as well as getting a lot of trouble with my nose, my eyes appear red and swollen and they water a great deal. They also feel itchy and sore. Can hayfever affect the eyes?

Yes. If you are allergic to pollen, it can cause problems in your nose, your chest and your eyes. The cause of all these problems is exactly the same: the pollen causes an allergic reaction which leads to inflammation.

Most people who have hayfever find that the eyes are affected as well as the nose, because the pollen grains can settle directly onto the surface of the eye. Inflammation of the most superficial layer of the eye is called conjunctivitis. Allergic conjunctivitis is much more common in younger people, and in at least 75% of the people who have it, it disappears by the age of 30.

In allergic conjunctivitis the eyes and eyelids can appear swollen, the eyes often look bloodshot, and itching and watering can also occur. In severe cases bright light feels uncomfortable, and there is an increased tendency to blink. Symptoms tend to be worst at the height of the pollen season, which can vary for individual plants.

Medications are available for allergies in the eye in the same way that they are available for nasal allergies. Although bathing the eye with solutions available from a pharmacy may help, the most effective medications are available only on prescription, so I would suggest that you see your doctor.

I wear contact lenses. I occasionally get eye infections, which my optician tells me are because of poor hygiene. However I am scrupulous about looking after my contact lenses and these infections only seem to occur during the hayfever season. Could they be caused by an allergy?

It is very important that you follow your optician's instructions on handling and cleaning your contact lenses, as eye infections due to poor hygiene can cause serious problems. However, the symptoms of a pollen allergy affecting the eye can be similar to those of an eye infection. If your symptoms always occur in both eyes simultaneously, then I would suspect that your problem is caused by an allergy, as it is very unlikely that a pollen allergy would affect only one of your eyes at a time. If only one eye is affected, then the most likely cause of your problem is infection.

The most important piece of advice remains the same, whether your problem is infection or allergy – stop wearing your contact lenses at once. If you continue wearing them, you will only make the problem worse. Ask your optician if she can see you while your symptoms are still obvious, as she may be able to tell you the cause of the problem after a careful examination of your eye. If it is an allergy, she could then refer you to your GP for appropriate treatment.

Triggers

What are pollens?

Pollens are small grains produced by plants as an essential part of the reproductive process. The pollen grains are the male seeds, which are light enough to be spread to other plants in order to pollinate or fertilise them. Although pollen grains are so small as to be invisible to the naked eye, they are potent allergens which can set off an allergic reaction in people who are already allergic to that type of pollen.

The pollens which cause the most severe allergic reactions are the ones which are carried from plant to plant by the wind, as these pollen grains are so light and dry that they can be carried in the air for many miles. The pollens from plants which are fertilised by insects tend to be larger and heavier, and are therefore less likely to be found circulating in the air.

I used to live in the country. Last year I moved because of my job and I now live in a city. I thought that this would be good for my hayfever but in fact since I have lived here it has been worse. Why is this?

Many people believe that living in a city should lead to an improvement in their hayfever. Unfortunately this is not true, for two reasons.

Firstly, pollen grains are very light and can be carried for long distances in the air. The number of pollen grains in the air (known as the pollen count) can therefore be just as high in a city as in the country. Most cities contain numerous parks and gardens, which means there are plentiful sources of pollen.

Secondly, although allergy to pollen is the primary cause of hayfever, it now seems that air pollution can also play a role, as air pollutants can irritate the lining of the nose causing it to become inflamed. Less pollen is then needed to start an attack of hayfever, and people with hayfever therefore seem to be more susceptible to inhaled pollens.

The government has introduced a new strategy to establish national air quality standards, and will be setting national limits for major air pollutants such as ozone, carbon monoxide, benzene, nitrogen oxides and sulphur dioxide. However these initiatives are in their infancy, and are unlikely to have a major impact for some time.

How do I know which type of pollen is causing my hayfever?

There are a number of tests available from your doctor which might be able to identify the culprit (they are described in Appendix 1). However, you might be able to pinpoint which pollen is causing your symptoms from the time of year at which they occur. These dates are approximate, as unusual weather conditions can advance or delay pollen seasons.

- The tree pollen season runs from late January to the end of June.
- The grass pollen season runs from April to September with a peak in June and early July.
- Oil seed rape flowers in May.
- Mould spores are found between May and October.
- Most weed pollens occur between the end of June and the beginning of September.

Sadly, even if you can identify which specific type of pollen is causing your problems, it will still be difficult for you to avoid it completely, because of the way that pollens are carried in the air. On the other hand, early treatment is the most effective: it should start two to four weeks BEFORE your symptoms appear. Once you know the pattern of your symptoms, you may be able to reduce them considerably in years to come by starting your hayfever treatment in good time.

I am allergic to grass pollen. Why, if the grass pollen season lasts for several months, are my symptoms so variable? On some days they are virtually absent whereas on other days I suffer badly.

Your symptoms vary because the amount of pollen in the air varies: they will be worse when the pollen count is high, and better when it is low. The pollen count is the number of pollen grains found in a cubic metre of air, and it can be profoundly affected by weather conditions. On hot days with little wind, the count is likely to be high, and it will rise throughout the day to reach a maximum by the late afternoon. A rain shower will have the effect of lowering the pollen count.

Air quality will also affect your symptoms, as high levels of pollutants in the air will exacerbate the effects of any given level of pollen. Your hayfever is probably at its very worst on those days when the pollen count is at its highest and the air quality at its lowest.

Pollen counts and air quality reports are produced daily and can be found in newspapers and on local television and radio programmes, when they are often included in the weather forecast.

I am troubled by itching and runniness of my nose and eyes, and these symptoms are similar to those of a friend of mine who suffers from hayfever. However, my symptoms don't seem to occur at any particular season, but happen all year round. Is this really hayfever?

As your symptoms are not seasonal, it is unlikely that they are caused by a pollen allergy. It does sound as if your problems are caused by an allergy of some kind, and the culprit is likely to be one of the allergens which is found throughout the year. In other words, you probably have perennial allergic rhinitis as opposed to seasonal allergic rhinitis, as discussed in the section on *Hayfever explained* at the beginning of this chapter.

In this country, the allergens which most commonly cause problems like yours are produced by the house dust mite and cats.

• House dust mites are minute creatures which live in soft furnishings, carpets and bedding, and which live off the human skin scales which we all shed all the time. It is the faeces (droppings) of these mites which contain the allergen which can be responsible for triggering symptoms of asthma, eczema and rhinitis. You will find more information about these mites in the section on *Triggers* in Chapter 1.

- The cat allergen is found in the animal's saliva. Because of the way that cats groom themselves, this allergen is spread widely over the cat's fur, from where it is transferred onto carpets, furnishings, and the hands and clothing of anyone handling the cat. This allergen can be responsible for triggering chest, skin and nose problems in susceptible people.

You need to work out which allergen is causing your problems: although it is most likely to be from cats or the house dust mite, it could be something else entirely. Your GP will be able to help you with this by taking a careful account of your symptoms, and perhaps by performing some tests (they are described in Appendix 1). You can then take steps to reduce your exposure to the allergen responsible (see the suggestions in the various sections on allergen avoidance in Chapter 9), which should help to reduce your symptoms. Your GP will be able to offer you effective treatment for any symptoms that remain.

Treatment

I know that there are plenty of medications that I can get from my doctor and from the chemist to help suppress the symptoms of my hayfever. If I can, though, I would like to use these as little as possible. Do you have any practical suggestions as to how I can try to control my symptoms without the use of drugs?

Firstly, I want to reassure you that all of the drugs available for the treatment of hayfever have been carefully researched and evaluated and, if used according to their instructions, are completely safe. However, I can understand your desire to do without them as much as possible. There are ways in which you can reduce your exposure to the allergens causing your symptoms and they are described in the various sections on allergen avoidance in Chapter 9. Reduced exposure means fewer symptoms, and fewer symptoms mean that you will need less treatment.

Are there medicines that I can buy from the chemist to treat my hayfever?

Yes, there are several quite effective medications which you can buy over the counter from your pharmacist without a prescription. However, please don't feel that hayfever is a such a trivial problem that your doctor would not think it worth treating. The symptoms of hayfever can have a profound effect upon your quality of life, and your GP will be pleased to help. A much wider range of treatments are available on prescription.

The following types of medication are available from your pharmacist without prescription, and they are all discussed in more detail elsewhere in this section.

• Antihistamines, in both tablet and liquid form.
• Decongestant tablets.
• Sodium cromoglycate nasal sprays (brand names include Rynacrom, Vividrin).
• Steroid nasal sprays (brand names include Beconase Hayfever, Syntaris Hayfever).
• Solutions for bathing the eyes.

Decongestant nasal sprays are also available, but these should not be used on a regular basis as they can lead to thinning and drying of the lining of the nose, and can therefore make your problem worse rather than better.

Do consult the pharmacist if you have any questions or concerns about using these medications and, in particular, if you are pregnant or breast feeding.

There are now so many remedies available for hayfever that I get confused. What is the best medicine for hayfever?

This rather depends on what your symptoms are. If you have sneezing and a runny nose, an antihistamine medication will help, but if you have a blocked nose, a steroid nasal spray will be more effective. These two different medications can safely be used in combination. Anti-allergy eye drops should be added if you have symptoms affecting your eyes. Commonsense measures, such as avoiding exposure to high levels of pollen (you will find suggestions for ways of doing this in Chapter 9) will also be helpful.

My friend and I both have hayfever. She swears by an antihistamine tablet that her doctor has given her. However, whenever I have tried using antihistamines, I have felt really sleepy and rather knocked out. Why is this?

In the past, the antihistamine preparations that were available were effective but had considerable side effects, the main one of which was to make people feel sleepy. Newer preparations have now been produced which do not have this side effect. I would suggest that you arrange to see your GP and ask for one of these non-sedating newer preparations, which include terfenadine (brand name Triludan), loratadine (Clarityn), astemizole (Hismanal) and cetirizine (Zirtek). Most of these preparations are only available on prescription, but it is now possible to buy some of them over the counter from your pharmacist.

If for any reason you continue to use a preparation which makes you feel sleepy, please remember that this can make it dangerous for you to drive a car or to operate any machinery, and that alcohol will make the sleepiness worse.

I used to use a nasal medication which came as an inhaler. My GP has recently changed my prescription and I have now been given a liquid nasal spray. Why is this?

For two reasons. Firstly, liquid preparations are distributed much more effectively in the nose, and are therefore better at treating the whole of the nasal lining. Secondly, until recently aerosol inhalers often contained CFCs (chlorofluorocarbons) which are known to be harmful to the atmosphere. All products produced in the European Union will soon have to be CFC-free: your new spray already is. I expect you will find that the new preparation works at least as well as, if not better than, your old one.

When you use your new spray, it is important that you use it correctly. You should lean forward so that your head is upside down and pump the spray into one nostril. Before you pump it again, briefly hold the spray the right way up so that it can refill.

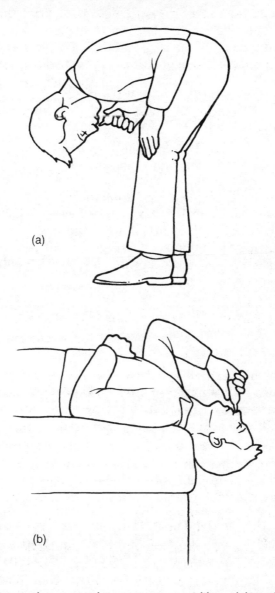

(a)

(b)

Figure 9: When using a nasal spray, you can either a) lean forward so that your head is upside down or b) lie on your back on the bed with your head hanging off the end of the bed.

Then treat the other nostril. If you find this position uncomfortable, lie on the bed on your back with your head hanging off the end of the bed, and then use the spray in the way already described. These positions are both shown in Figure 9.

In the past my hayfever has only affected my nose, but this year my eyes are itchy and sore all the time, and they run continuously. What can I do?

If you are not already taking antihistamine tablets (discussed earlier in this section), I would suggest that you start taking them. If antihistamines alone are not effective, you may find that anti-allergy eye drops such as those containing sodium cromoglycate (brand names include Hay-Crom Hay Fever, Opticrom Allergy and Vividrin) or a steroid preparation will help. Finally, bathing your eyes with a solution such as Optrex that you can buy from the chemists will wash away any pollen grains in contact with the eye and may be soothing.

In addition, it would be sensible for you to avoid going outside at times of day when the pollen count is high, and to try wearing glasses or sunglasses while you are outside. You will find more suggestions for reducing your exposure to pollen in Chapter 9.

My GP has prescribed eye drops for my hayfever, but he did not explain to me how I should use them. What is the best way of putting eye drops into my eye?

The easiest way is gently to pull your lower eyelid away from your eye and to place the drops into the space between your lower eyelid and your eyeball (as shown in Figure 10). When you blink, which will probably be immediately, the drops will then be spread over the whole surface of your eye.

None of the medications that my GP gives me for my hayfever is as effective as the decongestant spray that I can buy from my chemist. Why can't I just continue to use this nose spray?

Decongestant nasal sprays have an almost immediate effect and can make your nose feel much clearer. They work by decreasing the blood flow to the lining of the nose which, in the short term,

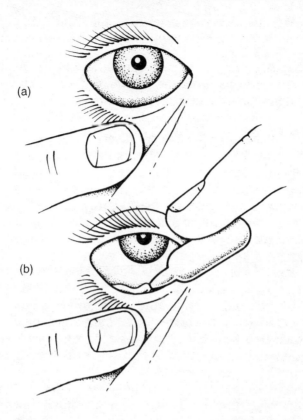

(a)

(b)

Figure 10: When using eye drops, a) gently pull your lower eyelid away from your eye and b) place the drops into the space between your lower eyelid and your eyeball.

reduces the swelling. However, if these preparations are used over a prolonged period of time, which means for more than a couple of days, they can lead to lasting damage, as the lining of the nose shrinks and dries out.

Decongestant tablets (which usually contain a combination of an antihistamine and a decongestant) do not cause this problem but again should not be relied upon long-term.

I know that the medications given to you by your doctor do not have an immediate beneficial effect but, if you persevere with them and take them as prescribed, they should relieve your symptoms without causing any damage.

My GP has told me not to use decongestant nose sprays for my hayfever and has instead prescribed me a steroid nasal spray. Surely these can have as many or more side effects than the old spray I was using?

Almost all medications have side effects, even the ones we take for granted such as aspirin and paracetamol. When doctors decide which drugs to prescribe, they have to weigh up the likely benefits against these side effects.

In the case of decongestant nasal sprays, the answer is clear cut. Prolonged use is always damaging to the nose (as explained in the answer to the previous question) and the beneficial effects are not long-lasting.

In the case of steroid sprays, the balance is very much in favour of the beneficial effects. The dose of steroid delivered by these sprays is extremely small, and very unlikely to have any generalised effect on the body. As they are given locally onto the part of the body where they are needed, they can therefore be given in sufficiently small doses that side effects are negligible.

Incidentally, the steroids that are used in these nasal sprays and in some anti-allergy eye drops are not the same as those abused by some athletes. Those are anabolic steroids; the ones used for hayfever are a different type called corticosteroids.

I recently went to my chemist to collect my prescription for the antibiotic that I take for acne, and to buy some more of my hayfever tablets. The pharmacist refused to sell me the antihistamines that I've been using up till now, because she said the combination of the two drugs was dangerous. Is this really true? What do I do about my antihistamines now as those were the only ones which didn't make me sleepy?

Sometimes taking two medications at the same time can cause side effects which do not occur if each medication is taken separately. One example of this is when the antihistamine terfenadine (brand name Triludan) is taken by someone who is also taking the antibiotic erythromycin (brand names include Erymax, Erythroped and Erythromid). In certain people this combination can cause heartbeat irregularities: although this problem is very rare, it is important that no one takes these two drugs together. You don't mention the names of the drugs involved in your case, but I suspect it was these two, and so your pharmacist was absolutely correct in what she did. To prevent anyone accidentally combining these drugs in the future, terfenadine has recently been made a prescription-only medication, so you will no longer be able to buy it over-the-counter at the chemist's.

Your problem about what to do about your antihistamines is easily solved by telling your GP about your hayfever symptoms and asking for a prescription for a non-sedating antihistamine which can be combined safely with the antibiotic you take for your acne.

Can hayfever treatment interfere with the contraceptive pill?

Whenever you are prescribed a new medication by your doctor, or buy a medication over the counter at the chemist, it is important that you tell the doctor or pharmacist about any other medications you are taking. So your concern is very sensible, but in this case I do not think you have anything to worry about. None of the antihistamine medications or the nasal sprays for hayfever affect the effectiveness of the contraceptive pill.

In the past when my hayfever was particularly bad, my GP used to give me an injection of something call Kenalog. This used to be very effective. My new GP is very reluctant to give me this. Why?

Kenalog is a steroid preparation which has a long duration of action and is given by injection. Steroid preparations can be very effective, but they can also have considerable side effects. In the case of steroid injections these include thinning of the bones, thinning of the skin and, in children, slower growth. In addition Kenalog can cause scarring at the site of the injection. If your hayfever can be controlled as effectively by using other medications such as steroid nasal sprays (which contain a much smaller dose than an injection) and antihistamine tablets, then this would be much safer for you in the long run.

I read that desensitizing injections can be very effective in hayfever. However my GP says that these are no longer available as they are dangerous. Is this true?

Desensitizing injections are no longer available in GPs' surgeries as a few people have suffered serious reactions to them, some of which have been fatal. This type of immunotherapy is still available in specialist hospital clinics, but tends to be reserved for serious allergic reactions such as those to bee and wasp stings. You will find more information about it in the section on *Allergy explained* in Chapter 1.

A newer type of immunotherapy is being tried for the treatment of hayfever. In this, the doses of allergen are given as a powder into the nose (the same way that the pollens enter the body), which means that injections are avoided. It is rather early to say whether or not this form of treatment is effective. Until we know, your hayfever is probably better treated by more conventional therapies such as antihistamine preparations and steroid nasal sprays.

Are there any complementary remedies that are likely to be helpful in my hayfever?

Homeopathic remedies containing eyebright (*Euphrasia officinalis*) or onion may be helpful. In addition, traditional herbal remedies which include garlic are thought to help hayfever and catarrh. Acupuncture has also been shown to be successful in both the prevention and the treatment of hayfever symptoms.

I discuss the place of complementary therapies in treating allergies in Chapter 9, where you will find more information on homeopathy, herbal medicine and acupuncture.

Living with hayfever

I like to go out for a walk each day. Is there a time of day which is least likely to provoke my hayfever?

The best times for you to be outdoors are early in the morning and in the late evening. During the day, the pollens produced by plants and trees are carried up into the atmosphere by warm air currents and therefore the pollen count rises, reaching a peak in the late afternoon and early evening. The air then begins to cool, and the pollen grains fall back down to earth.

You could also go out when it has been raining, as showers clear the air of pollen grains. If there is a rain shower in the afternoon or early evening, the air will then remain fairly clear of pollen grains until the following day.

I plan to have an early holiday this year which will be right in the middle of my hayfever season. Is there anything I can do to avoid a miserable holiday?

If you are planning a holiday in Britain, may I suggest that you try a seaside resort? Sea breezes often reduce the pollen count by the coast.

If you are planning a trip to Europe, I would suggest that you choose a country such as Greece or Turkey where the vegetation is very different from that in Britain. This would considerably reduce your chances of encountering the type of pollen which causes your hayfever.

If you have enough time and money to travel long distances, then a trip to the Southern hemisphere would almost certainly ensure you a symptom-free holiday, as instead of early summer it would be early winter there.

Wherever you go, make sure that you have sufficient supplies of your hayfever medications so that you can continue to take them throughout your holiday.

I drive a great deal in my job. Can I safely drive when I am using medicines for my hayfever?

You don't say what treatment you are taking for your hayfever, so

I can only answer in general terms. Nasal sprays and anti-allergy eye drops will not affect your ability to drive safely. Antihistamine tablets may: some of these medications cause drowsiness, whereas others do not. Most decongestant tablets contain a sedating antihistamine, so those might also make you drowsy. You should also realise that the symptoms of hayfever can themselves affect your ability to drive safely, so your best option is to take effective medication which does not have a sedative effect.

I suggest that you discuss your current treatment with your GP or pharmacist, remembering to tell them about the amount you have to drive. Most people whose work depends on a clean driving licence are extremely careful not to drink and drive, but it would also be sensible for you to ask if alcohol will alter the effects of your treatment. If you decide to try a new hayfever medication at any time in the future, then you should have the discussion again.

If you are able to choose what type of car you drive, consider changing to a model which has an integral pollen filter in the ventilation system to reduce your exposure to the allergens which trigger your hayfever. Unfortunately these filters have virtually no effect on chemical air pollution (they only remove

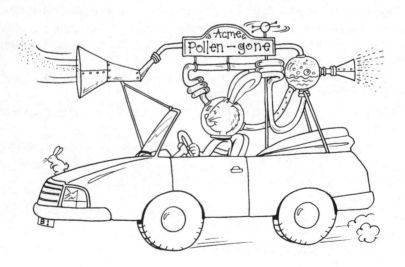

particles from the air), something to which you are invariably exposed when you drive a great deal and which can make hayfever worse.

I love gardening, but I get terrible hayfever! Do you have any tips to help me cope with my hayfever while I am in the garden?

Yes, and you will find them in Chapter 9 on *Allergen avoidance and complementary therapies*. I would also suggest that you see your GP, who may be able to give you some treatment which will considerably reduce your symptoms.

I am pregnant, and my hayfever seems a great deal worse. Why is this?

Pregnancy can have an effect on a number of medical conditions, including hayfever. In some women it gets better, in others it gets a great deal worse. However, your particular problem may have nothing to do with your hayfever. Many pregnant women experience a feeling of nasal obstruction during pregnancy, and this is thought to be due to a general increase in blood circulation, which can cause swelling in the lining of the nose.

I would suggest that you consult your GP, who will make sure you have the best possible treatment for your hayfever and that your medications are safe to continue during pregnancy. Unfortunately, as with many of the less-pleasant effects of pregnancy, it may be that this is something that you will have to put up with until after your baby is born.

Is it true that I shouldn't drink alcohol while I am taking antihistamines?

It is probably safest to limit your alcohol intake or to avoid alcohol altogether when you are taking antihistamine medications. You should be particularly careful about this if you are taking one of the older types (eg Piriton), as these can be quite sedating in themselves and can interact with alcohol to make you very drowsy indeed. The newer antihistamines – which include loratadine (Clarityn), astemizole (Hismanal) and cetirizine (Zirtek) – do not usually cause drowsiness, but it is still advisable not to combine them with alcohol.

In the summer I seem to lose my enjoyment of food. Is this because of my antihistamines?

No. Your hayfever itself will be the cause. The two senses of taste and smell are very closely related: in fact it is often the smell of food rather than its taste which gives it its appeal. You may have noticed that your food does not taste as good as usual when you have a cold and your nose is blocked. In the same way the smell of your food – and therefore its taste – is lost when your nose is blocked because of the effects of your hayfever. It sounds as if your antihistamines are not preventing all of your symptoms, and so you might benefit from a steroid nasal spray which can be prescribed for you by your GP.

My daughter seems to have a runny nose all year round. I have noticed that recently she seems to turn the volume on the TV up very loud. Could this be due to her allergy too?

Possibly. The nose and the ears are linked by small tubes called the Eustachian tubes, which are there to drain the middle ear and to equalise the pressure between the ears and the throat. The Eustachian tubes can become blocked if the nose and throat are inflamed, and an allergy can cause this inflammation. The blockage can cause fluid to collect in the middle of the ear, a condition called glue ear which can affect the hearing.

As even a minor degree of hearing loss can cause problems with schooling, I would suggest you take your daughter to your GP, who can prescribe medications which may help. If the problem continues, your daughter may need to be referred to an ear, nose and throat specialist for further treatment.

The skin around my nose and mouth gets very sore sometimes, especially when my nose is very runny. Is there anything I can do to stop this happening?

For immediate first aid, I suggest that you try putting petroleum jelly (eg Vaseline) onto the skin of your nose and lips first thing in the morning, and reapply it regularly during the day. To try and prevent this problem, you will need to go and see your GP, and ask whether there are any medications you could use to stop your nose running so much. You don't mention what treatment you currently use, but your hayfever sounds bad enough to warrant the use of both an oral antihistamine and a steroid nasal spray.

5
Food allergies

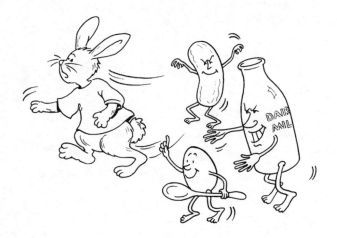

Introduction

Unpleasant reactions to foods are extremely common, but very few of them are due to allergy. The majority of people who have these reactions are not truly allergic to a particular food. Does this mean that they are imagining their symptoms? Of course not. Their symptoms are real and foodstuffs may, in some way, be responsible. However, I believe that it is important to make a clear distinction between true food allergy and the wide range of other unpleasant reactions which may be associated with food. In this book the term allergy is reserved for reactions involving the immune system in a particular way, as the treatment for a true allergy will often differ from the treatment of other, non-allergic reactions. People who wrongly attribute their symptoms to food allergy may be needlessly limiting their diet and their lifestyle.

This chapter will explain the difference between truc food allergy and the other reactions to food which can occur, such as food sensitivities and food intolerances. I hope it will help you to solve the puzzle of what is causing your problems. In some cases, factors other than food may be responsible for your symptoms, and it is important to recognise and to understand this so that these other issues – which include stress and anxiety – can be addressed. Sometimes it is not easy to discover whether an unpleasant reaction to food is caused by true allergy or by something else, but I think the effort is usually well worthwhile.

Food allergy explained

What exactly is food allergy? How common is it?

In this book I have used a very strict definition of allergy: an allergy is an abnormal or inappropriate reaction of the immune system to a substance which would normally be harmless, and involves the production of an allergy antibody called immunoglobulin E (this is discussed in more detail in the section on *Allergy explained* in Chapter 1). If you have a food allergy, then your immune system produces these antibodies each and every time you eat the food to which you are allergic, even when you only eat very small amounts of it. Using this definition, fewer than 5% of children and 1% of adults suffer from true food allergy.

However, as was discovered in a large questionnaire recently carried out in the United Kingdom, almost 10% of the population report that at some time in their lives they have had unpleasant reactions to specific foods, and almost 5% to food additives. A clinic was set up to investigate the people taking part in this survey who believed they had these allergies. When challenge tests using the suspected foodstuffs were performed, fewer than 1% gave positive results (there is more information about food challenge tests in the section on *Oral challenge tests* in Appendix 1).

There is therefore a wide discrepancy between the use of the word allergy by the general public and by the medical profession when it comes to describing food-induced reactions. These differences can matter, because if your problem is not correctly diagnosed you may not get the most appropriate and effective treatment for it. However, it might be that the only suitable treatment for your symptoms is to avoid the food which is affecting you, in which case it probably doesn't matter which term you choose to use.

If my symptoms are not due to a true food allergy, then what is causing them?

Apart from allergy, there are a number of different ways in which foodstuffs can produce unpleasant reactions.

- **Immunological disorders**
  A number of bowel diseases are caused by disorders of the immune system which make it produce antibodies other than immunoglobin E (there is more information about antibodies in the section on **Allergy explained** in Chapter 1). They include coeliac disease, which is discussed later in this chapter.

- **Food intolerance**
  If you are intolerant to a foodstuff, you develop symptoms after eating it because your body cannot adequately handle it. This is usually because your body does not produce enough of the particular chemical (enzyme) that is required for you to digest the food properly. For example, many Asian people feel ill after drinking even a small amount of alcohol because they lack the enzyme which breaks down the byproducts of alcohol. Similarly, some people cannot digest milk and milk products properly because they do not produce enough of the enzyme which breaks down cow's milk. For them, cow's milk in any

form causes crampy abdominal pain and diarrhoea. These two problems are not allergies, and they do not occur if only small quantities of the substance in question are consumed.

- **Food sensitivity**
  Some people find that an existing medical problem can be triggered by eating certain foods: they are then said to be sensitive to those foods. For example, some migraine sufferers find that red wine or cheese will provoke their headaches. Sufferers from irritable bowel syndrome (a problem which causes abdominal discomfort, diarrhoea and constipation) find that certain foodstuffs can make their problem worse. However, these foodstuffs are not the only cause of the problem in question, and these reactions are not allergies.

- **Food poisoning**
  This occurs when food contaminated with germs (bacteria or viruses) is eaten. Vomiting, diarrhoea and abdominal pain result.

- **Other possibilities**
  A great many people suffer a wide range of unpleasant symptoms which they themselves attribute to certain foodstuffs. Using the tests currently available, it is possible to determine in most cases whether a true food allergy is responsible or if the symptoms are due to a particular medical disorder. If the tests show that neither of these possibilities is the correct answer, it does not mean that the person is imagining that something is wrong with them. There is a great deal that we still do not know about how the body works and a large number of other factors – stress in particular – may be responsible for their symptoms.

You can see that blaming unpleasant symptoms on food allergy without proper medical advice could be dangerous, as the symptoms might be due to another illness that should be diagnosed and properly treated. In addition, if a food allergy is wrongly diagnosed as the cause of your symptoms, you might be tempted severely and unnecessarily to limit both your diet and your lifestyle. A balanced diet is essential for good health, and no foodstuff should be excluded from your diet without good reason. Whilst it is important that you avoid any food which triggers an unpleasant reaction, it is equally important to recognise and to understand that a number of other factors might explain your symptoms. I would recommend that you see your doctor, who should be able to arrange any tests you might need, and help you sort out the causes of your problem.

I am sure that I am allergic to a number of foods including sugar, wheat and several food colourings, but my GP does not agree. He has even gone so far as to describe my symptoms as psychosomatic. I am very angry about this, as I feel he is not taking me seriously, and is saying that I am neurotic. Can I organise a referral to a specialist myself?

I can understand why you are angry, as not only have you not been offered any help for your problems, you also feel insulted by what your GP has said. I doubt that he meant to imply that you were neurotic, but perhaps he could have offered more by way of explanation. I will try to fill in the gaps.

Firstly, foods associated with true food allergy are usually proteins. Wheat does contain protein, but sugar and food colourings do not, and these are rarely associated with food allergy. Sugars, which come in many different forms, are found in a huge variety of foods. They occur naturally in all fruits (where the sugar is called fructose) and dairy products (lactose). The majority of pre-prepared and convenience foods contain sugars (including sucrose, glucose, dextrose and maltodextrin). To avoid all foodstuffs containing sugar would limit your diet enormously. You can see that it is important for your problem to be diagnosed correctly, or you could find yourself eating a very limited and probably unhealthy diet. Your symptoms could be due to a wheat allergy, but again this must be formally diagnosed, because excluding wheat from your diet can also be complicated.

Secondly, although the term psychosomatic literally means 'of the mind and of the body' (it comes from two Greek words, 'psyche' meaning 'mind' and 'soma' meaning 'body'), it is more generally used to describe illnesses or disorders which are caused or aggravated by mental stress. It does not mean that you are neurotic, nor that you are imagining your symptoms. I do, however, feel that it is important that your general state of health and your lifestyle are taken into account when trying to diagnose what is causing your problem. Unpleasant reactions caused by food are not necessarily caused by an allergy (this was discussed in the answer to the previous question) and it is important for you to find out what is really causing your problem.

Finally, you ask if you can arrange a referral to a specialist yourself. In this country, that is not possible, nor do you have an absolute right to a second opinion. What the *Patient's Charter* (see Appendix 3 for how to obtain a copy) promises is the right 'to be referred to a consultant acceptable to you when your GP thinks it is necessary and to be referred for a second opinion if you and your GP agree this is desirable'. However, you do have the right to change your GP without giving a reason. You should think carefully about such a change, as there is no guarantee that a different doctor will take a different attitude, and there may be other things that you like about your current practice which you would be sorry to lose.

I think that your next move should be to go back to your current GP and try talking the matter through again. If you cannot resolve it between you, perhaps he will agree that you could see another doctor in the practice or will refer you to a specialist. If you are still dissatisfied after this, I would suggest that you get in touch with your local Community Health Council (the address and telephone number will be in your local phone book). The Community Health Council is an independent voice on health issues in the local community, and it also helps individuals like you who are unhappy with the care that they have received.

Why have I become allergic to just one or two foodstuffs and not to every food that I eat?

It is indeed amazing that food allergies are not more common, as the gastrointestinal tract is exposed to a huge number of substances which could potentially cause allergies. Although there is a great deal that we do not know about true food allergy, the fact that it is so rare demonstrates just how efficient the gut is at handling these potential troublemakers and in preventing the development of allergies in most people.

There are certain factors which might have made you more likely to develop a food allergy. You may come from an atopic family (atopy is discussed in the section on *Allergy explained* in Chapter 1) – does any other member of your family have an allergic disorder, particularly eczema? In addition, the way in which you were introduced to food in infancy appears to be important. Ask your mother how and when you were weaned (if she remembers) as this may throw some light on your pattern of allergies.

Food allergy appears to be less likely in babies who are breast-fed, particularly if certain foodstuffs are introduced into their diet later rather than sooner. These foodstuffs include cow's milk, eggs, peanuts, fish, and wheat and other cereals which contain a substance called gluten. Current Department of Health guidelines suggest that babies should be breast-fed or bottle-fed until they are at least 4 months old, and that other foods should then be introduced as follows.

- **At 4-6 months old**
  Vegetables, fruit other than citrus fruit, rice, meat, chicken and pulses (eg lentils).

- **At 6-12 months old**
  Foods containing wheat (eg pasta, bread, biscuits), fish, eggs, yoghurt, cheese and citrus fruit.

- **Over 12 months old**
  Ordinary cow's milk (ie milk straight from the bottle or carton as delivered by your milkman or bought from a supermarket).

Peanuts and foods containing peanut (including peanut butter) should ideally not be included in the diet until a baby is at least 12 months old, or until a child is 5 years old in atopic families where other family members have allergic disorders.

I am allergic to peanuts and to shellfish. I hope to have a baby in the near future. Is this type of food allergy inherited?

The tendency to develop allergic problems is called atopy and it is inherited, at least in part. As you yourself have allergies, any child of yours is more likely to be atopic than the children of parents who do not have allergies. This is discussed in more detail in the sections on *Allergy explained* and on *Inheritance* in Chapter 1.

However, whether or not an allergy develops is not simply a matter of inheritance. There are all sorts of other factors which come into play, some of which we know about, many of which I am sure remain to be discovered. Recent evidence suggests that an allergy is more likely to develop if certain foods such as cow's milk, eggs, wheat and peanuts are given at too early an age (current guidelines for introducing these foods into a baby's diet were given in the answer to the previous question). I would also strongly advise you to breast-feed your baby if possible, and you yourself should keep to a peanut-free and shellfish-free diet during your pregnancy.

Why is it that I have a severe seafood allergy yet my identical twin sister can eat whatever she likes?

You and your sister demonstrate beautifully the fact that, although inheritance is probably the most important factor in the development of allergy, many other factors also affect the process. You will both have inherited the same likelihood of developing atopy and allergy, but your life experiences will not have been identical. Something about the way you have come into contact with allergens (for example, how old you were at the time) has somehow led to you developing an allergy while your sister has not. This is discussed in more detail in the section on *Inheritance* in Chapter 1.

My doctor has diagnosed my 18-month-old son as being allergic to milk and eggs. Will this continue to be a problem for the rest of his life?

Allergy to milk and eggs is most common in young children, but fortunately it generally improves with age. If your son avoids eating milk and eggs for the next few years, then it is likely that he will become increasingly tolerant of them. By the time he is

4 or 5 years old he should be able to eat them without any problems. However, I would recommend you not to include milk and eggs in your son's diet until advised to do so by your doctor, and I would also suggest that he should be carefully monitored when these foodstuffs are reintroduced. In the meantime, you might find the advice of a dietician helpful in understanding how best to plan your son's diet to avoid these foodstuffs, and your GP can arrange this for you.

I am allergic to peanuts. Is it true that each time I inadvertently eat foods containing peanuts that my allergic reaction will get worse?

No, this is not necessarily so. Although you will have a reaction each time you are exposed to peanut, this will not necessarily get worse with each exposure. The severity of the reaction can be affected by other factors, such as stress and exercise. However, it is important that you remember that you will experience an allergic reaction each time: as these reactions can be severe you should ALWAYS avoid foods containing peanut.

Is food allergy becoming more common?

All allergies seem to be on the increase. This might simply be because we are more aware of and better informed about health matters these days. However, it does seem that there has been a real increase in the number of people suffering from food allergy and, in particular, allergy to peanuts. All food allergies are more common in people with a strong family history of the various allergic disorders (which include asthma, eczema and hayfever). Food allergies also appear to occur more frequently in the very young, when allergies to eggs and to cow's milk are common. As these allergies have usually disappeared by the age of five, food allergy is less common with increasing age.

It is not easy to calculate the actual number of people suffering from food allergy, as it is often difficult to work out whether an unpleasant reaction is caused by allergy to a foodstuff or by something else (this was discussed earlier in this section). In addition, many people with food allergy never go to see their doctor about their symptoms. The true size of the problem will emerge as more accurate methods of diagnosing food allergy become available and more accurate information is collected.

Is severe food allergy more common in men or women?

This problem seems to affect young males more than any other sector of the population. Of over a thousand people who have joined the recently formed Anaphylaxis Campaign (address in Appendix 2), 80% were under the age of 15, 85% were allergic to peanut, and the majority were male. Anaphylaxis is the most severe form of allergic reaction, and is discussed in more detail in Chapter 6.

I seem to read in the newspapers almost every day about somebody dying from severe allergies such as peanut allergy. As all of my family (I have three children) have allergies of some sort, including food allergies, I am terrified by this. How many people die from food allergies?

The chances of such a thing happening are extremely rare. In fact, the reason these deaths are reported in the newspapers is because they happen so rarely that they are therefore considered newsworthy. Some figures may help to put it in perspective. For example, we know that in this country approximately six people die each year from anaphylactic shock caused by bee and wasp stings (you will find more information about anaphylaxis in Chapter 6).

However, you specifically asked about deaths from food allergies, and here the most accurate information we have relates to peanut allergy. In the past year, only four people have died from anaphylactic shock after eating peanuts, although there may have been further deaths that were incorrectly diagnosed. One in every 500 adults and one in every 1000 children have an acute severe reaction to nuts each year, yet fewer than one in a million of these reactions will be fatal. Even people who have had a previous severe anaphylactic reaction have a greater chance of dying in a road traffic accident than of dying from their allergy. So although it is essential that allergic problems are taken seriously, please try not to worry unduly.

Symptoms

I am going abroad on holiday with a friend who is allergic to shellfish. I know she usually avoids eating them, but just in case she does so inadvertently, what should I look out for? What are the symptoms of food allergy?

Most allergic reactions due to food cause symptoms involving the gastrointestinal tract (the gut), and these symptoms begin when the food responsible comes into contact with the mouth. Tingling and itching of the lips and tongue, swelling of the lips and the lining of the mouth, and nausea and vomiting are all common. Food allergies can also produce symptoms in the skin, causing either urticaria or angioedema (both discussed in the section on *Skin allergies explained* in Chapter 3), and chest symptoms such as wheeziness and coughing. All of these symptoms usually occur within minutes of coming into contact with the food.

The most severe problem that can result from food allergy is called anaphylaxis. This is a potentially life-threatening reaction which involves the whole body. If untreated, it can lead to dizziness, shortness of breath, wheezing, palpitations, collapse and a serious drop in blood pressure. It is discussed in more detail in Chapter 6.

In some people the symptoms of food allergy do not occur immediately after eating the food, but only after a delay of several hours. This type of reaction is much more difficult to recognise. In addition, certain foods may make other allergic disorders such as asthma or eczema flare up.

You can see that the symptoms of food allergy can be very different in one person compared to another. They can also be different in the same person on different occasions. I suggest that you ask your friend for more information about her allergy: that way, you will know how best to help her. In general, however, you should remember the following points.

- Don't panic.
- Help your friend to take the medication she has been given to deal with an acute attack. This will usually be an antihistamine

but may also include an adrenaline injection (there is more information about this in the section on *Emergency treatment* in Chapter 6). Find out about her medication before you leave for your holiday.

- If the reaction appears to be getting worse and is causing her difficulty in breathing, dizziness, fainting or collapse, then call for immediate medical help.
- Even if her reaction responded well to treatment, if it was severe your friend should see a doctor as soon as possible.

How can I tell if my symptoms are caused by a food allergy?

This is often quite difficult even for the most experienced doctor! The following factors would make diagnosis of an allergy to a particular foodstuff more likely.

- Your medical history, in particular if you or other members of your family have other allergic disorders such as eczema, hayfever or asthma.
- A pattern of symptoms which occurs each time you eat a particular foodstuff.
- Symptoms which occur almost immediately after you eat that foodstuff.
- Symptoms which involve your gastrointestinal tract (your mouth, your gullet, your stomach and your bowels).
- Itching and swelling of your lips and mouth immediately after you eat that foodstuff.
- Symptoms which disappear when you eliminate the suspected foodstuff from your diet.

If you suspect that you have a food allergy, you should consult your doctor, who has a number of ways of diagnosing the problem. For example, you might be asked to keep a diary of your diet and your symptoms to see if there is a consistent relationship between the two, or you might have skin, blood or challenge tests to look for specific allergies. All these tests are discussed in more detail in Appendix 1.

If I am allergic to certain foods, how long after eating them can I expect to show symptoms of allergy?

In most cases of true food allergy, the symptoms occur almost immediately after eating the foodstuff responsible. The most common symptoms are swelling of the lips, tongue or face, difficulty in swallowing, abdominal cramps, nausea and vomiting.

In some cases, however, symptoms may not appear for several hours. In these cases, the symptoms are more commonly those of diarrhoea, abdominal pain, wheeziness, inflammation of the nose, and itchiness or inflammation of the skin.

Every case of food allergy is different, and it should never be diagnosed (or indeed ruled out) on the basis of the symptoms alone. A number of tests are now available which can help enormously in the diagnosis of your symptoms, and these can be organised for you by your GP.

Triggers

Is there a cure for food allergy?

No, there is no cure, so it is important for anyone with a true food allergy completely to avoid the food responsible. This may not be

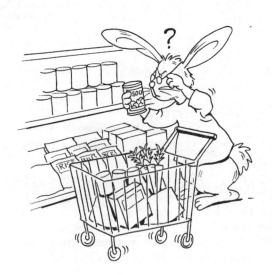

as simple as it sounds! Many of the foodstuffs responsible for allergy (particularly eggs, cow's milk and peanuts) are frequently used in the manufacture and preparation of foods, and their presence may not be at all obvious. You will therefore have to scrutinise all labels on prepared foods, and carefully question waiters and chefs when you go to restaurants to make sure that the food causing your allergy isn't in the dish you wish to eat.

Some anomalies in the way foods are labelled will make your task even more difficult.

- **The 25% cut-off rule**
  Present EU regulations state that any item which itself consists of more than one ingredient does not have to have the component ingredients of each product it contains listed if that product makes up less than 25% of the overall food. This rule sounds complicated, but what it means is that items such as salami used as a pizza topping or sponge fingers contained within a trifle would not have to have their individual component ingredients listed on the packaging.

- **Vegetable oils**
  Under present rulings, vegetable oils can be identified on a food label simply as that, rather than giving the specific name of the oil being used, such as peanut oil (also called groundnut oil) or corn oil. This means that if you are allergic to peanuts, you will have to avoid ALL foodstuffs labelled as containing vegetable oil to be certain of avoiding peanut oil.

Finally, you need to be aware that certain allergens can crop up in the most surprising places. For example, at least one multivitamin liquid contains peanut oil, and almond oil can be found in brands of antiseptic creams and depilatory creams. If you have a severe allergy and are ever in any doubt about a product, then do not use it until you have checked it with your pharmacist or directly with the manufacturer.

I think I may have developed an allergy to something I eat, but I don't know what. Which are the most common foodstuffs to trigger allergic reactions?

You are much more likely to be allergic to some foods than others, and which these are depends somewhat on your age. The commonest food allergies in infancy are to cow's milk and egg. Other food allergies can develop at any age, with the most common being to peanuts (which are actually not nuts at all – they are legumes, belonging to the same family as peas and beans), true nuts, shellfish, white fish, soya beans, wheat, corn, bananas and citrus fruit.

Sometimes it sounds as if everything you eat can cause an allergy. Are there any foods which don't?

Foods which are rarely responsible for allergies include the following.

- **Fruits**
  Apples, grapes, peaches, pears, plums.

- **Meats**
  Lamb, turkey.

- **Vegetables**
  Carrots, potatoes, rice, green beans, the squash family (which includes courgettes and marrows).

- **Grains**
  Barley, oats, rye (although these all contain gluten, and must be avoided if you have coeliac disease, which is discussed later in this chapter).

If I am allergic to a food does that mean that I should never eat it?

This rather depends upon how severe your allergy is, how difficult that particular food is to avoid, and how much you like it. If your allergy is so severe that every time you eat a particular food you end up in hospital, then obviously you would be wise never to eat it. On the other hand, if your reaction is mild and perhaps limited to urticaria (nettle rash, discussed in the section on *Skin allergies explained* in Chapter 3), you will do yourself no serious harm if you eat the food occasionally. It's up to you to decide whether it's worth the itching!

The way in which a food is prepared may make a difference to your reaction, particularly in the case of protein foods such as milk and eggs. For example, some people find that if they eat raw eggs (perhaps in mayonnaise or ice cream) they develop an allergic reaction, which they do not have when they eat cooked eggs. Similarly, milk drunk in its natural form may cause an allergic reaction, whereas cooked milk (eg in a rice pudding) does not. This is because the process of cooking denatures the protein in the food, ie alters it in a way which means that it is no longer such a potent allergen.

I am allergic to nuts – my symptoms include swelling of the lips, tingling inside my mouth and nettle rash. I have heard that if I avoid nuts for a year or so my allergy will disappear. Is this true?

No. Generally speaking, once you have developed an allergy, your immune system maintains a memory of the responsible allergen in the form of antibodies, and the allergy is therefore lifelong (this is discussed in more detail in the section on *Allergy explained* in Chapter 1). The main exception to this is when an allergy develops in early childhood – as the immune system is then rather immature, its memory is not quite as good. Therefore children who are allergic to substances such as cow's milk and eggs in the first few years of life often outgrow their allergies. However, as you grow older, you may find that your allergy becomes less active, although you would be wise to continue to avoid nuts in your diet.

I believe that the peanut is not actually a nut. Why then, now that I have been diagnosed as having peanut allergy, have I been advised to avoid all other nuts as well?

You are right: peanuts are a legume (they belong to the same family as peas and beans) and not a true nut (sometimes called tree nuts to distinguish them from the peanut or groundnut). Being allergic to peanuts does not automatically mean that you will be allergic to other nuts, although some people do have both allergies. However, peanuts are often used as a cheap substitute for other more expensive nuts, as they can be washed to remove the peanut flavour and then treated so as to taste like something else – walnuts or brazil nuts, for example. The nut inside your hazelnut chocolate may actually be a peanut! It is for this reason that you have been advised to avoid ALL nut products, although if all your tests to true nuts were negative, it would be safe for you to eat them providing you remove them from the shells yourself and therefore know EXACTLY what you are eating.

I recently had a moderately severe reaction to walnut, so my GP arranged for me to have some tests, which showed that I am also allergic to almonds. Are these nuts related?

Multiple nut allergies are relatively common, as there are chemical similarities between the different types of nut. People who are allergic to walnuts are often allergic to almonds as well. Similarly pistachio nut and cashew nut allergies often go together.

Occasionally, people with a food allergy may develop a reaction to other closely-related foods. Groups of these closely-related foods include the following examples.

• Barley, corn, oats, millet, rye, black-eyed peas, liquorice, lima beans, peas, pinto beans, green beans such as French beans and runner beans.
• Blackberries, loganberries, raspberries, tayberries, strawberries, cashew nuts, pistachio nuts, mango.
• Chocolate, cocoa, cola.
• Grapefruit, lemons, limes, oranges, tangerines.
• Peaches, plums, cherries, almonds, apricots.
• Crabs, crayfish, lobster, langoustines, scampi, shrimp, squid.

How come I am very allergic to peanuts but not to any other members of the legume family?

Although there are chemical similarities between foods in the same food group, no two foods have exactly the same chemical structure. It is therefore possible to be allergic to one food but not to another with a similar but not identical chemical make-up. For example, by no means all people with peanut allergy react to other legumes – in fact, this is relatively unusual.

My child is allergic to milk. Can he eat beef?

Yes, he should have no problem eating beef. The proteins found in milk are not found in the muscle tissue of beef meat, which can therefore be eaten without provoking an allergy.

My baby daughter is allergic to eggs. I am concerned about her having the MMR vaccine which I believe is grown on egg. Will this be a problem?

If your child is truly allergic to hen's egg, and this has been confirmed by skin prick testing, you are right to be cautious. Some makes of the MMR (measles, mumps, rubella) vaccine can contain a minute trace of egg protein, and this can, in very rare instances, be enough to cause an allergic reaction. It would be sensible to make sure that your doctor knows that your daughter is allergic to egg so that he can check that the vaccine used is egg-free.

If her egg allergy produces severe symptoms, then she will need to be skin prick tested to the vaccine before vaccination. If no response occurs, the vaccine can then be given safely. The skin prick testing should be done by someone expert in the technique, and the vaccination by someone trained and equipped to deal with the very small chance that your daughter might experience a reaction. This means that both steps should be done in hospital.

Please don't be put off this vaccination, or indeed any of the other vaccinations offered to small children. None of the other vaccines contain egg protein, and in the case of the MMR vaccine, even taking into account her egg allergy, the risks to your daughter of the diseases themselves are much greater than those of the vaccination.

Diagnosis

I think I am allergic to preservatives and food colourings, which seem to make me moody and tired. How should I go about finding out if I'm right and which of them is the problem?

At the beginning of this chapter I made a clear distinction between true food allergy and other reactions to food which caused people problems. I think it is unlikely that your symptoms are due to a true food allergy, but it is possible that you could be reacting in some way to food colourings and preservatives. It is hard to believe that all those E numbers can be good for you!

Product labelling has improved a great deal over recent years, and you will now find it far easier than it used to be to see which foodstuffs contain which E numbers. Information about which additives may cause problems and which foods contain them is available from the major supermarkets. You may find leaflets about them in your local branch, or you may need to write to the head office for them (your local branch will be able to give you the address).

I think your first step should be to avoid all food colourings and preservatives for a period of two weeks by eating only fresh food, and to see whether your symptoms improve. If they do, it would be worthwhile asking your doctor for a referral to a dietician, who might be able to identify the culprits and to give you advice on avoiding them. If your symptoms are unchanged during this trial period, then you should arrange to see your doctor for a thorough check-up, as other problems such as anaemia can cause the type of symptoms you are experiencing.

I think that eating milk and eggs makes my 3-year-old son's eczema worse. How can we prove this, as I don't want to change his diet unless it will be worthwhile?

You are very wise to want to find out whether or not your son is allergic to milk and eggs before you exclude them from his diet. At his age they are important for good nutrition, and it would be time-consuming and potentially bad for his overall health to exclude them from his diet unless absolutely necessary.

I suggest that you arrange to see your doctor, who will be able to choose the best way to find out whether your son has a food allergy. The following tests are discussed in more detail in Appendix 1.

- **Skin prick testing**
  This is the most commonly used allergy test. It only takes
  about 15 minutes and may provide much useful information.

- **RAST**
  This can be a more accurate test than skin prick testing but it
  does involve taking a blood sample.

- **Symptom diary**
  Also called a food diary, this is simply a record of what your
  son eats and how bad his eczema is, and it is used to see if
  there is any relationship between the two. It might be
  worthwhile starting this two weeks before you go to see the
  doctor and taking it with you.

Sometimes the only way to see whether a particular foodstuff is
making a condition like eczema worse is to exclude it from the
diet and see what happens. This should only be done under
medical supervision, especially when children are involved. If
you were to put your son on an exclusion diet without proper
advice he could end up eating a diet containing too little of those
foodstuffs which are essential for his good health and his proper
growth.

**I think I am allergic to something in my diet, as I keep on
getting swollen lips and nettle rash, but neither my doctor
nor I can work out what food is responsible. What can I do?**

Diagnosing food allergy can be extremely difficult, especially if
you have no clues as to what it is that is causing the trouble. I
think your first step should be to ask your GP to refer you to an
allergy specialist. While you are waiting to see the specialist, you
should keep a food diary (also called a symptom diary). The diary
should be a detailed record of everything that you have eaten
over a period of several weeks, and you should also note down
any symptoms you had during that time. Comparing your diet and
your symptoms will give the specialist useful clues to the possible
cause of your problems.

Your GP may already have arranged for you to have skin prick
tests or blood tests to see if these will help identify the allergen

responsible, but if not, the specialist will be able to do this. However, these tests may not give you the answer, as a positive skin test can be produced by a food which does not cause symptoms when eaten, and blood tests are not always 100% accurate.

Your specialist may then suggest an elimination diet (sometimes called an exclusion diet). Under your doctor's supervision, you would remove from your diet those foods likely to be the culprits, to see if your symptoms disappear. If they do, you then reintroduce the foods one at a time, with an interval of at least three days between foods. If your symptoms reappear after introducing a particular food, you have found the cause of your problem.

The final stage of diagnosis is to perform a food challenge. The best way to do this is so that neither you nor your specialist knows what foodstuff you are being given: this means that the results of the challenge cannot be prejudiced by the expectations of either one of you. You will be given a capsule, which may contain an extract of the food suspected of causing your allergic reaction, or which may contain no active ingredient at all. Even your doctor will not know at this stage: someone else will keep the records of what you have been given. If no reaction occurs when you take a particular food capsule, then that food cannot be blamed for your allergic symptoms. On the other hand, if your symptoms of nettle rash and swollen lips come on after eating a particular food (even though you didn't know you were eating it, because of its disguised form), then you are sure to have found the cause.

All the tests mentioned here are discussed in more detail in Appendix 1.

I recently experienced a severe allergic reaction to a food which we haven't, as yet, identified. My GP wants to arrange allergy testing for me but I am frightened that I might react badly to the skin prick tests. Are they safe?

Skin prick testing (explained in detail in Appendix 1) is part of the standard investigation of an allergic problem, and the more severe that problem, the more important it is that the cause be identified. The tests are safe and painless, although a positive reaction will produce an itchy red bump (weal) on your forearm which can last for an hour or so.

It is extremely unlikely that you will have a dangerous reaction to skin prick testing. If you do (this is very rare), please be reassured that the person performing the test will have available to them all the resources necessary to treat the reaction immediately, and that you will come to no harm.

My daughter was recently skin prick tested to a number of different substances when she attended the asthma clinic at our local hospital. I was surprised to see that she had a positive reaction to testing with egg, as she has never shown any signs of egg allergy. Does this mean that she now has to avoid eating eggs?

If we skin prick tested the whole population of the United Kingdom, we would find that approximately 40% would show at least one positive reaction to an allergen, although only one-third of these people would have clear-cut symptoms of allergy. It is not surprising that your daughter had a positive skin test, as most people with asthma have a tendency towards allergy (for more information about this, see the sections on *Allergy explained* in Chapter 1 and *Asthma and allergy* in Chapter 2). Providing that she has never had symptoms of allergy after eating eggs and that her asthma is well controlled, I would suggest that she should continue to eat a full, normal diet.

There is more information about skin prick tests in Appendix 1.

When he was 9 months old, my son became very swollen around the face and had wheezy breathing after eating food containing peanut. Since then we have avoided peanut completely in his food. He is now 2 years old. My GP has suggested that we now try him with a small amount of peanut butter to see if he really is allergic to peanuts. Do you think that this is a safe thing to do?

Allergy to peanuts often appears in early life, and for most people it remains a lifelong problem. For many years, doctors kept track of a group of people who had peanut allergy: all of them were still allergic to peanuts 16 years after they were first diagnosed. I would therefore suggest that you continue to exclude peanut from your son's diet. If at some time in the future you or your doctor want to find out if he is still allergic to peanut, then skin prick testing would be the first step. If these tests were negative, they could be followed by a small dose of peanut – but this peanut challenge test should be done in hospital.

The tests mentioned in this answer are discussed in more detail in Appendix 1.

My local supermarket has started running an allergy testing service. Apparently a small sample of blood is taken by pricking your finger and the results of up to 12 allergy tests are sent to you in the post. How accurate is this type of testing and is it worth the money?

Advances in modern technology now mean that a relatively large number of allergy tests can be performed on a small sample of blood – it is a form of multiple RAST (RAST is explained in Appendix 1). Providing the tests are done by a reputable laboratory, there is no reason why they should not be accurate, but that is not the whole point. The results of blood tests like these will not, in themselves, give you adequate information to enable you to diagnose and manage any allergies which you may have, as all tests of this type must be interpreted in the light of your clinical symptoms (ie those you can describe or which your doctor can observe). As this interpretation can only be done by a trained doctor, I would advise you against using this service.

Living with food allergies

My 4-year-old daughter has a severe cow's milk allergy, which not only gives her vomiting and a rash, but which also makes her eczema and her asthma much worse. I am hoping to have another child. If I completely avoid cow's

milk in my own diet during my pregnancy and during breast-feeding, will my next child avoid this allergy?

You are very sensible to think ahead about how you can decrease the chances of your next child developing allergies. You are right in thinking that he or she will be more at risk of developing an allergy in the light of your daughter's current problems. However, allergies do not necessarily run true within a family (see the section on *Inheritance* in Chapter 1 for the reasons why) and your next child could be completely well or could become allergic to something other than cow's milk. This partly depends on to what degree your child inherits a tendency towards atopy, something which is passed on from both the father and the mother.

It may well be worthwhile thinking about avoiding cow's milk during your pregnancy and while you are breast-feeding. Some foodstuffs (and milk is one of them) can pass across the placenta to the unborn baby in the womb and can also appear in breast milk in sufficient amounts to cause a baby to become allergic to them. I think that your own GP or your daughter's specialist would be the best people to help you decide whether avoiding milk is a good idea for you in your particular circumstances. It is not an easy undertaking, and you will need help from a dietician to make sure that you eat a diet adequate in calcium and protein.

There are a number of other ideas that you could discuss with your doctor. While you are pregnant, you could reduce your exposure to other common allergens such as the house dust mite, and cat and dog dander (the scales from their hair or fur, something like dandruff in humans), and avoid all exposure to tobacco smoke. Once your baby is born, you could avoid introducing those foods known to trigger allergies into his or her diet until as late as possible. The foods most likely to be responsible are discussed in the section on *Triggers* earlier in this chapter, and you will find information on allergen avoidance in Chapter 9.

I never let my two small children eat peanuts because of the danger of them choking. Shortly after I myself had eaten some peanuts the other day, I noticed that my son

had developed swelling of the lips. I had just given him a kiss and a cuddle. Could this really have been caused by the tiny amount of peanut from my lips?

Once someone has developed an allergy to peanuts, if it is severe they can develop a reaction just from touching a peanut to their lip or, as in your son's case, being kissed by someone who has been eating peanuts. It sounds to me as though your son may well have a severe peanut allergy, and he should be tested for this as soon as possible. This can be done either by a simple blood test or by skin prick testing, both of which can easily be organised by your GP (you will find information about these tests in Appendix 1). I suggest you do this without delay, and that in the meantime you make sure that your son avoids all contact with peanut.

I suspected that I was suffering from a food allergy and, having received no help from my GP, I consulted an alternative practitioner. He suggested an elimination diet, and I have been eating only boiled chicken, rice and pears for about three weeks now. I am getting very bored with this, and also quite hungry! Is it safe for me to go back to a normal diet?

I personally feel that complementary practitioners and their skills have a lot to offer, and that in certain conditions they can provide some very effective therapies. I discuss this further in the section on *Complementary therapies* in Chapter 9. However, this does not mean that I automatically think that they always offer the correct treatment!

In your case it sounds as if you have been subjected to a very strict exclusion diet, and I am seriously concerned about the adequacy of your current diet. Extreme elimination diets should only be introduced under careful medical supervision, and usually require the help of a skilled dietician. If your alternative practitioner has immediate plans for reintroducing you to a normal diet, then by all means go along with this. If he does not, it is essential that you return to a more balanced diet immediately, although you may wish to exclude a small number of foodstuffs if you are very suspicious that they may be the cause of your problems. I think you need urgent help, so I suggest that your next move should be to go back to your current GP and try talking the matter through again. If you cannot resolve it between you, perhaps he will agree that you can see another doctor in the practice or will refer you to a specialist.

My husband has asthma and when he takes his medication (ie if he remembers!), his symptoms are well controlled. I have recently been diagnosed as being allergic to sesame seeds and I am disappointed that, instead of being offered treatment for this allergy, I have just been told to avoid eating sesame seeds. Why is this?

The only way to make absolutely sure that you do not experience an allergic reaction to sesame seeds is not to eat them. In other words, there is no effective treatment for food allergy: the mainstay of management is avoiding the problem foodstuff. However, you may well find that it is useful for you to keep a supply of antihistamine tablets to hand for the occasions when you accidentally eat sesame seeds.

If your food allergy was severe, for example if it caused breathing difficulties or anaphylactic shock, you would have been supplied with a drug called adrenaline. This can be given by injection from one of two special injection kits; you will find more information about their use in Chapter 6, which deals with anaphylaxis. Treatment with adrenaline is not necessary in mild cases of allergy.

In the very rare cases where someone has multiple severe food allergies, an anti-inflammatory drug called sodium cromoglycate (which is sometimes used in asthma) can be given in very large doses by mouth in an attempt to damp down the allergic reaction. This treatment is reserved for very serious allergies, and sadly it is not always effective.

My 2-year-old daughter has been diagnosed a having an allergy to egg, and we have been advised to exclude all egg-containing foods from her diet. I am finding this much more difficult than I had thought, as egg seems to be everywhere! Do I have to avoid all prepared food?

I am sorry you are finding this so difficult, although I am not really surprised. Once you start looking, it is amazing just how many foods seem to contain egg. Most cakes, biscuits, chocolates, soups, sauces, custards, ice creams, pancakes, sweet breads, pastries and batters contain egg, and you will soon develop a sixth sense regarding which foods you should avoid, although it is always best to check the label as well. When checking labels, be aware that egg can go by several different names, including albumen and egg white.

Something you might find especially helpful is a list of packaged or prepared foods which are free from egg. These lists can be obtained from all the major supermarkets – if your local branch does not have one, write to the head office (the branch will be able to give you the address). Having such a list to hand will mean that you will not be forced into cooking every meal from scratch. Be aware, however, that sometimes manufacturers change the formulations of processed foods. If one of your favourite standbys is described as 'new' or 'improved', check the label to make sure that egg has not suddenly been included. In your daughter's case, new might not necessary mean improved.

You might also find it helpful to speak to a dietician about your daughter's diet – ask your GP, who will be able to arrange a referral for you.

I am allergic to peanuts, and just recently I have noticed that a large number of foodstuffs in my local supermarket have started carrying labels stating that they may contain traces of peanuts. I am confused – these are foods which I thought were peanut-free. Is it safe for me to eat them or not?

The large supermarket chains have become increasingly aware of the problem of peanut allergy, and are trying their best to make sure that people with this allergy can confidently identify which foods they should not eat. The foods which are labelled as possibly containing traces of peanut do not themselves have peanut as an ingredient, but may have become contaminated during the manufacturing process with sufficient peanut protein to cause an allergic reaction. This can happen, for example, when a batch of jam doughnuts are moved on a conveyor belt which has previously been used for peanut biscuits. If your peanut allergy is severe, it would be safest for you to avoid all these foods. Although this might mean that your choice is more restricted, the good news is that you can be confident that the remaining foods are safe for you to eat.

I have several food allergies, but I love eating out. This obviously poses problems. How can I be certain of avoiding problem foods?

There is no way of being completely certain that the food you are eating is free of a particular ingredient unless you have made the food yourself from start to finish. Foodstuffs such as peanut are widely used in food preparation and often appear in the most unlikely dishes, such as lemon meringue pie and Chinese spring rolls.

Depending upon which foods cause your allergy, it might be possible to choose a style of restaurant which is less likely to cause you problems. For example, if you are allergic to peanuts, you should avoid Chinese, Thai and Malaysian cuisines, as they rely very heavily upon this ingredient. Whichever type of restaurant you choose, and however careful you are to choose foods which do not contain your problem foodstuffs, you should remember that it is still possible for one dish to become

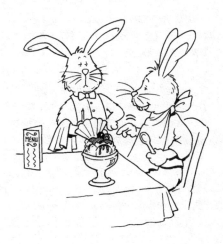

contaminated with an ingredient from another. For example, meat could be cooked in a pan which had previously contained fish.

As you enjoy eating out so much, I would advise you to become a frequent visitor to a small number of restaurants where you feel you can trust the staff to take your allergy seriously, so that you know that they will answer your questions about ingredients honestly. If you have to eat out in a strange restaurant when you are away from home, you should choose simple dishes and, if possible, see the chef yourself to explain your allergy.

I only seem to be allergic to soya-containing foods in the summer. Why is this?

This does seem strange at first sight, but I think I can explain it. Firstly, it might be that for some reason you eat more soya-containing foods in the summer, making what is otherwise a mild allergy flare up. Secondly, one allergy can be made worse by another: it might be that you suffer from hayfever, and so during the hayfever season you find that you become more sensitive to soya.

Coeliac disease

My 5-year-old daughter has been getting terrible diarrhoea, and is very thin. My GP thinks that this could be due to coeliac disease. What is coeliac disease? Is it due to an allergy?

Coeliac disease is a problem of the small intestine caused by an intolerance to a protein called gluten, which is found in wheat, rye and barley. The word 'coeliac' simply means 'relating to the abdomen' and comes originally from the Greek word 'koiliakos' which means 'belly'. Coeliac disease is also known as gluten-sensitive enteropathy: 'enteropathy' means 'disease of the bowel' and again the word comes from the Greek (from 'enteron' meaning 'gut' and 'pathos' meaning 'suffering').

The problem is not an allergy in the way that I have defined allergy in this book: the IgE antibody is not involved. However, the immune system certainly is involved and antibodies of the IgG and IgA types are found in the blood streams of a significant number of people who have coeliac disease. You will find more information on all these antibodies in the section on *Allergy explained* in Chapter 1.

It certainly sounds possible that your daughter could have coeliac disease. Sufferers often lose weight and diarrhoea is common, as the reaction to gluten damages the lining of the bowel wall, making it less able to absorb water and nutrients from the food within it.

Although a doctor may suspect coeliac disease from your daughter's symptoms and her medical history, further tests will be required. A blood test will show if there are any anti-gluten antibodies in her blood stream, but the only way to confirm the diagnosis is to perform a bowel biopsy (as described in Appendix 1). It is very important to make a definite diagnosis by biopsy as treatment involves lifelong avoidance of all foodstuffs containing gluten, something that we would not want to impose on anyone unless it was absolutely necessary.

I suffer from coeliac disease, and am finding it extremely difficult to buy gluten-free bread and cakes that are worth eating – most of them are disgusting! Can you help?

There are approximately 100,000 gluten- and wheat-sensitive people in the United Kingdom, but sadly none of the major supermarkets sell gluten-free bread and cakes. They are available – as are gluten-free biscuits, bread mix, pasta and flour – at most health food shops, at many large chemists, and from specialist suppliers whose details can be obtained from the Coeliac Society (address in Appendix 2). These products are improving all the time, but whether or not you enjoy them is a matter of taste.

As you obviously do not like the commercially-available products, one answer might be to bake your own using gluten-free flour, although it is difficult to reproduce the texture of normal bread and cakes as gluten provides elasticity and fluffiness. As alternatives you could try using rice flour, potato flour or maize flour, all of which are available from health food shops.

If you have proven coeliac disease, gluten-free foods (including flour) can be prescribed on the NHS. Your GP can arrange this.

I have been diagnosed as having coeliac disease, but despite eliminating all wheat-containing foods from my diet, my symptoms have not got much better. What am I doing wrong?

Firstly, you should be aware that gluten is found not only in wheat, but also in rye, oats and barley. You should therefore exclude all four of these cereals from your diet.

Secondly, you may still be eating gluten-containing foods without realising it. Many foods list starch as an ingredient – but you have no way of knowing whether or not this starch is made from wheat. In theory, you should avoid all foods containing starch.

Avoiding all these foods can be very difficult, but help is now at hand. The Coeliac Society (address in Appendix 2) maintains a list of gluten-free foods produced by all major manufacturers. Most of the major supermarkets can now provide information about gluten-free foods produced under their own brand names: if your local branch does not have the list, write to the head office for it (the branch will be able to give you the address).

6
Anaphylaxis

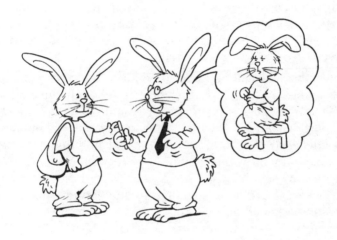

Introduction

Anaphylaxis is the most severe of all the allergic reactions, but fortunately very few people with allergies or allergic disorders will ever experience it. Those of you who have never suffered such a reaction probably never will. However, this chapter should be read by everyone, as one day the information it contains may help you to save someone else's life.

If you yourself have experienced an anaphylactic reaction,

then this chapter will give you an understanding of why it happened and what can be done to prevent it happening again. I hope this knowledge will help you to be less frightened and to lead as normal a life as possible. Your friends and family, colleagues at work and holiday travelling companions might also find it useful.

Anaphylaxis explained

I only heard of anaphylaxis for the first time fairly recently, so I looked it up in my dictionary – but that left me none the wiser! Please can you explain what it involves?

In common with all allergic reactions, anaphylaxis happens because you are exposed to an allergen to which you are allergic. The reaction is severe, even life-threatening, and is not confined to the part of your body which the allergen touches: it can affect the whole body. The most dramatic and potentially dangerous symptoms of anaphylaxis include swelling and obstruction of the upper airway, severe wheeziness, and failure of the circulatory system to work efficiently, leading to shock and collapse. If you suffer an anaphylactic reaction you will need urgent attention – first aid initially, and then afterwards in hospital.

Although this type of reaction can be extremely dangerous, if it is recognised promptly and treated effectively you will recover completely with no lasting damage. If you have suffered one anaphylactic reaction, you are at risk of further similar reactions. You can see that it is vital that the allergen responsible is identified so that you can do your very best to avoid it in the future. However careful you are you can never be completely sure of avoiding a particular allergen, so it is also important that you are provided by your doctor with effective emergency treatment. You will have to learn how to use this treatment correctly, and so will your friends and family.

The word anaphylaxis comes from two Greek words: 'ana-' meaning 'again' and 'phylaxis' meaning 'guarding' or 'protection'.

As anaphylaxis cannot happen the first time you are exposed to an allergen, we could roughly translate the word as meaning 'to guard again' against a second or subsequent exposure to the allergen concerned.

My friend has recently come out of hospital after an anaphylactic reaction to a bee sting. It sounds as if the whole thing was terrifying. She felt so ill that she can't remember exactly what happened, so can you tell me what happened to her?

Anaphylaxis is a sudden allergic response which can vary in severity, but which is often serious. I am sorry that this happened to your friend, but very pleased to hear that she, like most people, responded well to treatment and has now recovered.

In your friend's case a bee sting was responsible, but anaphylactic reactions can also be triggered by other forms of insect stings, and by foodstuffs (especially peanuts and shellfish), drugs (especially penicillin and certain other antibiotics) and vaccines (particularly the tetanus and diphtheria vaccines).

After the bee stung her, your friend would probably have begun to feel unwell very quickly. The symptoms that she might have experienced include:

- a feeling that something awful was about to happen;
- a flushed face;
- a red raised itchy rash ;
- sneezing, nasal congestion (a stuffy nose), itching in the mouth;
- palpitations;
- a feeling of being uncomfortably hot;
- dizziness;
- nausea, vomiting, abdominal cramps;
- shortness of breath;
- tightness in the chest, wheezing;
- swelling of the lips, tongue and face; and
- shock and collapse.

Your friend may not have experienced all of these, as every person's reaction is different, and the parts of the body affected also vary from individual to individual. If the reaction was particularly severe, your friend may have lost consciousness. It is also possible that she may have had severe breathing problems, and even that her heart might have stopped.

Now that your friend knows she is at risk of anaphylactic reactions she should always carry with her a ready-to-give adrenaline preparation, as described in the section on *Emergency treatment* later in this chapter. She should also wear some form of identification to warn others that she has this problem, and this is discussed in the *Miscellaneous* section in Chapter 8.

I have had several bee stings in the past, but last year was stung again and suffered an anaphylactic reaction. Why did this suddenly happen?

For someone to suffer an anaphylactic reaction to a particular allergen they must have been sensitized to it as a result of a previous exposure. In your case, you have been sensitized to the allergen in bee venom by being stung many times in the past – but why you suddenly reacted so severely to this latest sting is impossible to explain. As yet no one knows why an allergen which was previously not a problem should trigger an anaphylactic reaction, nor why an 'ordinary' allergic reaction can suddenly become something much more serious.

Now that you have had one anaphylactic reaction, you should assume that all further bee stings will lead to equally severe reactions. You should try to avoid being stung, and you will find some suggestions on how to do this in the section on *Living with anaphylaxis* later in this chapter. You should also ask your doctor to supply you with a suitable adrenaline preparation and teach you how and when to use it: you will again find more about this later in this chapter, this time in the section on *Emergency treatment*.

My son recently had the most awful anaphylactic reaction after eating food containing peanuts. Why did the reaction affect his whole body and not just his mouth and stomach?

Your son is so allergic to peanuts that eating a food that

contained them caused his body to react strongly, producing a huge amount of a number of different chemical substances. These substances were then rapidly spread throughout his body by his blood stream (that is why more than just his mouth and stomach were affected). They acted on the small blood vessels in his body tissues and made them leak, which in turn caused swelling. The effect of this leaking and swelling is different in different parts of the body: in the lungs it causes wheezing and breathing difficulties; in the skin it causes redness, itching and blotchy patches; in the bowels it causes nausea and stomach cramps. All the organs in the body can be affected in anaphylaxis – the heart as well as the lungs, skin and bowels.

Because an anaphylactic reaction is so widespread, enough fluid can leak out of the small blood vessels to reduce the total volume of blood circulating around the body. Once this happens, blood pressure drops and the heart finds it difficult to pump hard enough to maintain an adequate blood supply to the vital organs. This is why faintness, dizziness and even loss of consciousness can result. As you saw, this can happen extremely quickly, and only tiny amounts of an allergen are needed to set off this type of reaction. It is vital to recognise the seriousness of this type of reaction and to act quickly, as you undoubtedly did in your son's case. The sooner treatment is given, the more quickly these effects can be reversed.

How do I know if I am at risk from anaphylactic shock?

You don't, until you have had your first anaphylactic reaction. I realise that this sounds very harsh, but we have no way of knowing which individuals will be vulnerable or when such a reaction may happen. However, we do know that people who have asthma, hayfever or other allergic disorders are at greater risk of anaphylaxis from most causes than those who have never had an allergy. Bee and wasp stings are the exception – anaphylaxis can occur in individuals with no previous history of allergic problems.

Have you had any severe allergic reactions in the past? If you have, and in particular if they involved angioedema (discussed in the section on *Skin allergies explained* in Chapter 3), then you would be wise to see your doctor. Your GP will be able to arrange for you to see an allergy specialist, who will review your medical history and advise you whether or not you need to carry adrenaline. The use of adrenaline is discussed in the section on *Emergency treatment* later in this chapter.

Until a year or so ago I had never heard of anaphylaxis, but now I seem to be reading about people dying from it all the time. Just how common is this?

The chances of such a thing happening are extremely rare. Severe allergic reactions are becoming more common, and the general public are becoming more aware that they can be a serious problem, but the reason these deaths are reported in the newspapers is because they happen so rarely that they are therefore considered newsworthy.

Some figures may help to put it in perspective. We know that in this country approximately six people die each year from anaphylactic shock caused by bee and wasp stings. In the past year, only four people have died from anaphylactic shock after eating peanuts, although there may have been one or two further deaths that were incorrectly diagnosed. Although this is a small number, it is still too many, as every death from anaphylaxis is potentially preventable.

Greater public awareness about the causes and the treatment of this problem is essential if death is to be avoided, so the media coverage is perhaps no bad thing. However, it is important to keep worries about the risks in proportion. Although each death is tragic for the family concerned (especially as young fit people are generally those affected), in reality your chances of dying are extremely small. Even people who have had a previous severe anaphylactic reaction have a greater chance of dying in a road traffic accident than of dying from their allergy.

Could cot-death be due to anaphylaxis?

The cause of cot-death (the medical name is sudden infant death syndrome, sometimes abbreviated to SIDS) is not known. We do not believe that anaphylaxis is involved, but allergy may well be a contributing factor in the sudden death of previously well infants, and is one of the many possible causes under investigation. Although we still do not know why cot-death happens, thankfully the number of cases has fallen recently by over one-third. This is since parents have been advised to encourage their infants to sleep on their backs or on their sides, not their fronts.

Emergency treatment

My 12-year-old son was admitted to hospital recently with an anaphylactic reaction caused by a wasp sting. When he left hospital we were given an adrenaline emergency kit and told what to do in case it happens again. But I was so relieved that he was better that I don't think I took in all the first aid instructions properly. Please can you tell me what I'm supposed to do?

I am glad to hear that your son has recovered. You had a frightening experience, so it is not surprising that you did not take in everything you were told at the time. I hope you never have to go through it again, but the following advice will be helpful should it unfortunately happen.

The most effective way to prevent your son having a similar reaction in the future is for him to avoid being stung again by a wasp, and there is some advice on this in the section on *Living with anaphylaxis* later in this chapter. However, it is impossible completely to eliminate the risk of wasp stings, which is why your son must carry his injectable adrenaline with him at all times. He should learn how to give himself the injection, as it is possible that he could be stung when alone. It is also important that several members of your family and some of the teachers at his school also know how to give the injection, just in case he is unable to do it for himself for some reason.

If your son is stung by a wasp again, this is what you must do.

- Try to stay calm.
- Give him a dose of injectable adrenaline according to the

instructions. I suggest you familiarise yourself with these now by reading the instruction leaflet with the kit, and by asking your doctor or nurse about anything you do not understand.

- Get immediate medical help, which will usually mean dialling 999 and asking for an ambulance. Tell the ambulance control that your son is known to have a severe allergy and carries adrenaline, so that they understand that the problem could be serious.
- While you are waiting for the ambulance to arrive, get your son to lie down, as this will help to restore his blood pressure.

Do not delay in doing any of these things. It is far better that you overreact than act too late. There will be no harmful effects if you give a dose of adrenaline when it is not strictly necessary, so administer it if you think your son is beginning to have a severe reaction. Do not wait until you are sure, as that could be too late. In all of the recent deaths from anaphylaxis in this country, adrenaline has either not been given at all or has not been administered in time.

Make sure that you periodically check the expiry date on the adrenaline emergency kit to make sure that it will be effective if your son needs it.

It is possible that your son was also given some tablets to take in the case of another severe reaction. These could be either antihistamines or steroids. Whichever they are, on their own they will not be enough to treat a severe reaction: your son must always have the adrenaline first.

Can an adrenaline injection do me any harm?

Adrenaline is a hormone (chemical messenger) which we all have in our bodies, and we produce it every time we exercise or are under stress or are scared. It has been used as a drug for over 100 years, and it was once widely used in the treatment of asthma attacks. Because of its long history, it is a very well-understood drug and we know that it is very reliable.

I know nothing about you, but unless you are very elderly or have a heart condition there is no need for you to be worried about the effects of an adrenaline injection. All it will do is to push your heart rate up to the sort of level it would reach if you had just been playing sport. However, in someone having an anaphylactic reaction, a dose of adrenaline could be enough to save their life.

Can people who hate needles and injections have their adrenaline in a different form?

No, not if they are at risk of anaphylaxis. Giving adrenaline by injection is currently the only effective way of administering adrenaline for the treatment of severe allergic reactions.

It may help you overcome your dislike of needles if you remember that adrenaline injections can be life-saving. The idea of giving yourself an injection is very much worse than the reality, and with a little practice most people overcome their fears. The Epipen (shown in Figure 11) is the most commonly prescribed adrenaline injection. It has a pre-filled syringe and a spring-loaded needle you can't even see, and these features make it very easy to use. You take off the cap, and firmly press the tip of the Epipen against the side of your thigh. There is no need to take off your clothes. An alternative but similar device is called the Anapen. Nurses at a specialist clinic will teach you how to use your adrenaline, and I am sure that you will soon become an expert.

Incidentally, the name Epipen derives from the American word for adrenaline, which is epinephrine.

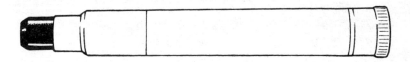

Figure 11: Epipen.

I had an awful reaction to shellfish once; my lips and tongue became very swollen and I felt quite wheezy. My GP gave me two sorts of tablets and an inhaler called Medihaler-Epi to use if the symptoms happened again. I've had a letter from my GP saying that I can no longer use the Medihaler-Epi, and to make an appointment to be taught

how to give myself adrenaline injections. I am horrified! Why can't I use the Medihaler-Epi?

It sounds as if you had an allergic reaction which was quite severe and extremely unpleasant, but not severe enough to be classified as an anaphylactic reaction. Your GP prescribed you the appropriate treatment for this type of reaction, which was antihistamine and steroid tablets, and an adrenaline inhaler called the Medihaler-Epi.

Unfortunately, although the Medihaler-Epi was a very simple way of administering a small dose of adrenaline which could be absorbed from the lungs, it has been shown to be inconsistent in the dose that is delivered by each puff. So it has been withdrawn by the manufacturer and all patients previously using the Medihaler-Epi will now be prescribed an injectable form of adrenaline.

You will have to be taught how to use the adrenaline injection. I can understand if you feel frightened, as an inhaler seems much less threatening than an injection. Please be reassured that using an adrenaline injection kit is not the same as giving an injection with a syringe and a needle (see the answer to the previous question).

You should use your adrenaline injection as soon as you experience any of the symptoms that suggest you might be getting another severe allergic reaction. Your GP will probably have given you a detailed treatment plan, which may look something like this:

- use your adrenaline injector (Epipen or Anapen) as you have been taught;
- take one dose of the antihistamine tablets you've been given;
- if the reaction is severe, take one dose of your steroid tablets;
- continue taking the antihistamine and steroid tablets for three days if your reaction was particularly severe.

If your symptoms do not begin to subside after one injection, seek medical attention at once, if necessary by calling an ambulance.

I have been given an adrenaline injector to carry with me at all times after suffering an anaphylactic reaction to peanuts. How do I know when to use it?

However hard you try to avoid eating peanuts, you may one day inadvertently eat peanut-containing food and begin to develop a severe allergic reaction. You should give yourself an injection of adrenaline at the very first symptoms that suggest that you might be developing such a reaction. Do not wait until you are certain. It is far better to give adrenaline unnecessarily than to give it too late.

It is best to give the injection in your thigh, half way between your knee and your hip. It is not necessary for you to undress, as the injection can be given through your clothes, providing they are not too bulky. Try not to be embarrassed about the idea of giving yourself an injection in public: most people these days have heard about peanut allergy, and will be extremely sympathetic. Once you have given the injection of adrenaline you should seek medical advice.

It is important that you become familiar with the equipment and comfortable with the idea of giving yourself an injection, so that when the time comes you do not hesitate. A trainer kit with an inactive liquid inside is available for practice sessions, and your doctor or nurse will be able to show you exactly what to do.

I have had several anaphylactic reactions in the past, but the most recent reaction I had responded very well to the adrenaline injection. Is it really necessary for me to go to the casualty department as last time they kept me waiting for hours and I was perfectly okay?

Severe allergic reactions are not predictable, and although your next one could be minor, it could also be more severe. Adrenaline is a short-acting drug, and its effects can wear off after 10 minutes or so. It is therefore advisable for you to be observed for several hours by medically trained staff who can assess your need for any further treatment. As you have suffered from anaphylaxis in the past, you should treat every allergic reaction you experience with great respect.

You should never drive yourself to the hospital, as there is the risk that the adrenaline could wear off while you were in charge of the car and that you could suffer a relapse. This would be dangerous for other road users as well as for you.

Identifying the cause

What allergens most commonly cause anaphylactic reactions?

Wasp or bee stings and peanuts are the most common triggers, followed by true nuts, shellfish, fish, eggs and penicillin. Once you have suffered an anaphylactic reaction, you should assume that your allergy is lifelong, and should always avoid the substance that triggers it.

Do bee and wasp stings always cause anaphylactic reactions?

No. Only a small minority of people (fewer than 1%) will ever develop this form of severe reaction. Everyone who is stung by a wasp or a bee will experience some discomfort at the site of the sting, and this can vary from a small amount of swelling with redness and tenderness to quite extensive swelling with considerable pain. These are not symptoms of an allergy, but occur because the sting contains an irritant. First aid is usually all that is needed – the following points are useful to remember if you are stung.

- Keep calm and do not run.
- If you were stung by a bee, the sting will often remain embedded in your skin (wasps do not leave their stings behind). Try to remove the sting with tweezers without squeezing it, as that will release more of the irritant.
- Keep the affected part cool and, if possible, apply an icepack.
- If the pain is considerable, take a mild painkiller such as aspirin, paracetamol or ibuprofen.
- If the swelling is severe, take an antihistamine (available from a pharmacist).

An anaphylactic reaction cannot occur the first time you are stung, but may occur on any subsequent sting. Once you have developed anaphylaxis, you will always experience a serious reaction if stung again, and so you should try, wherever possible, to reduce your risks of being stung. There are some suggestions on how you can do this in the section on *Living with anaphylaxis* later in this chapter.

I have now had two anaphylactic reactions to peanuts. Am I likely to react in a similar way to anything else?

You would be extremely unlucky if you did. Most people who suffer anaphylactic reactions do so to only one allergen, and that allergen can usually be identified. If you feel yourself developing the symptoms of anaphylaxis, don't waste time thinking about what might have caused it: start treatment immediately.

I recently suffered my first anaphylactic reaction to peanuts contained in a dessert. Why, if my doctor knows what caused this reaction, do I now have to go through a load of tests?

It is useful to know the cause of any allergy, as this makes management of the problem so much easier. This is particularly true of anaphylaxis. You and your doctor need to be 100% confident about the cause of your reaction, so that you can do everything possible to avoid a further exposure. After all, the dessert you ate probably contained other things besides peanuts, and one of them might have been the culprit.

The tests which your doctor will arrange are completely safe and really quite simple. You will find more information about all of them in Appendix 1.

- **Skin prick testing**
  You will be tested with a range of allergens, including peanuts. A positive response to the peanut allergen does not necessarily identify peanut as the culprit, but a negative test would rule it out.

- **RAST**
  A small sample of blood is examined for specific allergy antibodies. If peanut was the cause of your reaction, you are likely to show a positive result from this test.

- **Challenge test (oral provocation test)**
  Most allergy clinics no longer perform challenge tests for the

diagnosis of anaphylaxis as they can be dangerous, and adequate information can usually be obtained from other forms of tests. However, if your skin prick test and RAST both gave negative results as far as peanut was concerned, a specialist might decide on a challenge test. This would be done very cautiously, in a different way from that used for diagnosing non-anaphylactic food allergy (the double-blind food challenge test described in Appendix 1). The specialist would begin by putting a small amount of peanut on your lip, and would then wait 15 minutes to see if there was any reaction. Increasing amounts of peanut would then be put in your mouth, again with the wait of 15 minutes between each step. If this test was completely negative, then you could be sure that peanut was not the cause of your reaction, and the true cause could then be tracked down.

An advantage of skin prick tests and RAST is that other allergies sometimes associated with peanut allergy (such as walnut allergy) can be identified.

My son recently suffered an anaphylactic reaction for the first time after eating in a Chinese restaurant. We had chosen a wide range of dishes, including a fish dish, so we have no idea what it was that caused his reaction. I am now incredibly nervous about giving him anything other than very plain and simple food to eat. How can we find out what caused his reaction?

The three most likely foodstuffs to have caused his reaction are peanut (which is found frequently in Chinese and other Asian food), shellfish (which might have been contained in the fish dish or in fried rice) and white fish.

It is vital that your son is seen by an allergy specialist so that he can undergo a full range of tests to diagnose his allergy. He will have skin prick tests and RAST (both of which are described in Appendix 1), and from these it should be possible to pinpoint the culprit. In the meantime it is important that he has injectable adrenaline to hand at all times in case he has a further reaction (the use of adrenaline was described in the previous section on *Emergency treatment*).

Please ask your GP to arrange a referral to an allergy specialist as soon as possible.

I saw my doctor write 'idiopathic anaphylaxis' on my medical notes. What does this mean?

Usually the cause of anaphylaxis is obvious as the reaction follows an insect sting, or the administration of a drug to which someone is allergic, or it comes on after eating a particular food. However, in your case your doctor has been unable to identify what caused your anaphylactic reaction, and the trigger remains a mystery. Hence the description 'idiopathic', which simply means 'of unknown cause' (it comes from two Greek words, 'idios' meaning own and 'pathos' meaning suffering). This puts you in a very difficult situation, as you know that you have a potentially life-threatening problem but do not know what causes it.

It is essential that you do two things. Firstly, you must carry an emergency adrenaline injection kit (eg an Epipen) with you at all times, and you should treat any future reaction as early as possible (you will find more information about this in the previous section on *Emergency treatment*). Once you have given yourself an injection of adrenaline, you should always seek emergency medical attention. Secondly, you should make a very careful record of all the possible trigger factors with which you came into contact in the hours before your reaction. I hope that you do not suffer any more severe reactions in the future, but if you do, the cause may become clearer and therefore easier to avoid.

I have an allergy to shellfish. In the past any reaction that I have had has been relatively mild, and confined to a little swelling of my lips and some tingling in my mouth. I have to admit that I have not been scrupulous about avoiding seafood. The other day I finished a small quantity of my flatmate's Chinese takeaway and then went out for a long run. The next thing I remember I was in hospital having had a severe anaphylactic reaction. Why did this happen?

It sounds as if you suffer from a relatively unusual problem called food-dependent exercise-induced anaphylaxis. Exercise can act as a co-factor (an additional trigger) in anaphylaxis: if you eat shellfish you suffer only a mild reaction, if you exercise you have no reaction at all, but if you eat shellfish and then exercise you develop an anaphylactic reaction. The exercise appears to potentiate (strengthen) the allergic reaction, although no one is exactly sure how or why this happens.

It is important that your shellfish allergy is confirmed by skin and blood tests (they are described in Appendix 1). Once you know exactly what caused your severe allergic reaction, it is vital that you avoid this foodstuff completely in the future. You will then be able to exercise without worrying.

Living with anaphylaxis

I am allergic to peanuts and my last reaction was severe. I ended up in hospital. How can I avoid similar reactions in the future?

As you have now had one serious anaphylactic reaction, you must assume that your problem is life-long, and do all that you can to minimise the risk of further reactions.

- **Be vigilant about all the foods you eat**
  Educate yourself about what you are eating and read the labels like a detective, looking for the hidden peanut. Whole peanuts are obvious, but peanut can be included in a wide range of prepared and cooked foodstuffs, and may be described on labels as 'groundnut' or 'arachis'. Ask yourself what the exact source of the vegetable oil or hydrolysed vegetable protein listed on the label might be – it could be peanut.

  Restaurants can pose a particular problem, as waiters and chefs might not understand how important your questions are. You might find that fast food chains suit you better, as they have strict quality control and list their ingredients for you to check.

- **Ask for information**
  Do not be embarrassed or apologetic about asking for detailed information from restaurants and food manufacturers. The more pressure we exert on them to provide accurate detailed ingredient lists the better.

- **Know about adrenaline injections**
  Make sure that you are completely comfortable with the administration of the adrenaline kit you have been prescribed (the section on *Emergency treatment* earlier in this chapter may help with this). Ask if you can have a dummy kit to practice with. Make sure that other people around you know how to use it. Don't be frightened of adrenaline: the dose you will give yourself has very few side effects, and is completely safe.

- **Write an action plan**
  Get together with your doctor and your family and write an action plan for how to handle an emergency. Have several copies of this: carry one in your pocket, and leave others where they can be seen, for example in the kitchen at home and in your office at work. Check that everyone knows where your adrenaline is kept and make sure that they would be prepared to use it in an emergency.

- **Be alert to all symptoms**
  Give yourself adrenaline even if you have only the hint of a suspicion that you might be beginning to develop a severe reaction. Do not wait until it is too late. Get to hospital as soon as possible, making sure that someone else drives you, or call for an ambulance.

- **Tell other people**
  Be open about your problem with your workmates, friends and family. It is not something to be ashamed or embarrassed about. The more people who know about it, the safer you will be.

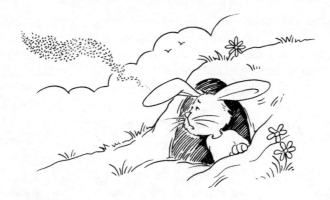

I am allergic to bee stings, and the last time I was stung I had an anaphylactic reaction. My doctor has prescribed me an Epipen but has told me the best treatment is to avoid being stung. Does this mean that I have to lock myself indoors for the whole of the summer?

You were unlucky to have suffered anaphylactic shock from a bee sting, and I can understand that you now must be very nervous about being stung again. Try to remember that bee stings are relatively rare, and that these insects only sting when provoked. Bees are not naturally aggressive, and once they sting they die.

I would hate to think of you locking yourself away for the summer! If you pay attention to the following pieces of commonsense advice, your chances of being stung will be small. I suggest you avoid wasps as well as bees, just in case you prove to be allergic to the stings of both, something which is relatively common. Honey bees generally nest in commercial hives, but other types of bees and wasps can build their nests anywhere.

- Never disturb stinging insects' nests or hives.
- Stay away from areas that attract insects, such as gardens, picnic grounds, and the areas around dustbins and litter bins.
- Keep dustbin areas and patios clean.
- Get someone else to mow the lawn and trim the hedges.
- Don't walk barefoot out of doors.

- Avoid wearing perfume and any cosmetic preparations with strong fragrances, as these smells attract insects.
- Wear plain light-coloured clothing, because bright colours and patterns attract insects.
- Avoid loose-fitting clothes, as insects could become trapped inside them.
- Keep your car windows closed if possible, and make sure that no bees or wasps are inside your car before you get in.

Even with all these precautions it is impossible completely to eliminate the risk of bee stings so you should, of course, always carry your Epipen with you just in case. There is more information about Epipens in the section on *Emergency treatment* earlier in this chapter. I would also suggest that you wear a piece of identification jewellery stating that you are allergic to bee stings, and you will find details of how to obtain this in the *Miscellaneous* section in Chapter 8.

My son has now had two very bad reactions to wasp stings, and I am told that he almost died the last time he was stung. I am now so terrified that I can hardly bear to let him leave the house in summer. I have heard about desensitization, and have asked my doctor if he could arrange this, but he tells me that it is no longer performed. I would do anything to cure my son of his problem. Is there anywhere that I can go to arrange desensitization treatment?

Desensitization (allergen immunotherapy) is a form of treatment in which repeated injections of very small amounts of allergen are given. The aim is to reduce the person's allergic responsiveness to that particular allergen. This form of treatment was widely used in this country in the past, but in 1986 the government put stringent restrictions on its use, because there had been increasing numbers of severe adverse reactions, including some deaths. It can no longer be performed by GPs, and specialist allergy clinics can only carry it out if they follow very detailed guidelines.

A recent document prepared by a working party of the British

Society for Allergy and Clinical Immunology summarised the benefits and risks of desensitization. They recommended that this form of treatment does have a place, but only in certain selected groups of people. You are right in thinking that desensitization can be extremely useful in wasp and bee sting-induced anaphylaxis. However, it is important that the benefits outweigh the risks, and in the case of children, this is not usually so.

Your son has been unlucky to be stung twice, and it may be many years before he is stung again. Even if he did undergo desensitization treatment, the benefits might not be long-lasting: the effects might have worn off by the time he was stung again. Although desensitization is always carried out in hospital and is always performed by doctors who are fully trained in the treatment of any problems which might arise, there is still the risk of the treatment itself causing a severe reaction (which would be extremely unpleasant for your son). Overall, I feel that the advice that you have received is correct, and that your son should not have desensitization treatment.

Please don't despair! There are a number of commonsense precautions that you can take to reduce the chances of your son being stung again (see the answer to the previous question). In addition, he should always carry injectable adrenaline with him in case of a further sting (there is more about this in the section on *Emergency treatment* earlier in this chapter), and I think that he should also wear an identification bracelet stating that he is allergic to wasp stings (details of how to obtain these are in the *Miscellaneous* section in Chapter 8).

The best news of all is that your son has a good chance, perhaps as high as one in two, of growing out of his allergy. I am sure that when he is older his specialist would be happy to test him using either RAST or skin prick testing (both described in Appendix 1) to see whether his allergy has gone.

I recently suffered an anaphylactic reaction after a shot of penicillin given by my dentist for a tooth abscess. Luckily he had all the right equipment to treat my reaction, and he acted very promptly. I am now very anxious about

receiving any drug treatment, especially antibiotics, and I am petrified about ever having to have another injection. What are the chances that I will have another similar reaction?

The cause of your anaphylactic reaction seem quite clear – it was the penicillin which was responsible. Further doses of penicillin could cause the same thing to happen again, so it is essential that you avoid it in all its forms for the time being. A number of different drugs belong to the penicillin family: not only penicillin itself but also cloxacillin, flucloxacillin, ampicillin, amoxycillin and azlocillin. They are available under a wide number of trade names, including Amoxil, Augmentin, Floxapen, Magnapen, Penbritin and Timentin. You should avoid all of these, whether they are given as injections, tablets, capsules, liquids or creams.

Fortunately there are plenty of other antibiotics available which are completely different from the members of the penicillin family. You will not be allergic to these, so your doctor or dentist should have no problem in choosing a safe antibiotic for you when you next need treatment. There are a few illnesses which are still best treated with penicillin, but the good news is that penicillin allergy tends to wear off with time. If it was ever essential to treat you with penicillin in the future, you could be skin prick tested to see if you were still allergic to it (this test is described in Appendix 1). However, for now you should avoid it.

You can see that it is essential for you to inform your doctor and your pharmacist that you are allergic to all forms of penicillin. You might find it helpful to register with a service such as Boots Medilink: your allergy will be recorded on their database and all medications (whether on prescription or bought over the counter) will be checked to make sure they are safe for you. Your local pharmacist may offer a similar service.

7
Allergies at work

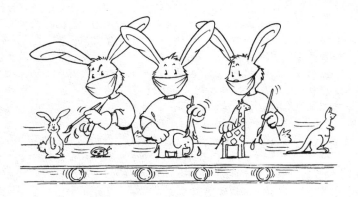

Introduction

We have known for hundreds of years that certain health problems can be associated with certain jobs. For a long time, however, little attention was paid to this link, as the more onerous and dangerous jobs were done by slaves or prisoners, whose lives were felt to be expendable! The first Government Act relating to working conditions in this country was passed in 1802, and since then numerous Acts have followed to try to ensure that employees' working conditions are safe. Although we have made great advances in this area, there are still a large number of health problems – some of which are allergic in origin – which are caused by contact with certain substances (more properly called allergic sensitizers) during the working day. As you can spend about one-third of your life at work, this makes it a significant cause for concern. When investigating an allergic problem, doctors should always ask you about your work.

You don't have to be atopic to develop a workplace (occupational) allergy. Although an hereditary predisposition to asthma, eczema or hayfever makes you slightly more likely to develop a workplace allergy, most of these problems occur in people with no previous history of allergy. Some of the problem substances you come into contact with at work might not cause allergy, but act as irritants instead: an important difference, for two reasons. Firstly, it is much easier to protect yourself from the irritant effects of a substance than to deal with an allergy once it has developed; and secondly, you are only eligible for compensation if a true allergy can be demonstrated. Because of these two points, this chapter concentrates on true allergies, rather than including all unpleasant reactions to substances met in the workplace.

There are over 200 substances which can act as allergic sensitizers causing occupational asthma, and at least an equal number causing skin allergies. It is therefore impossible for me to cover every single substance in this chapter, but I hope to provide you with enough general information to help you recognise whether or not your problem might be caused by a substance found in your workplace. The various types of allergy mentioned here are all discussed in greater detail elsewhere in this book (eg asthma in Chapter 2 and dermatitis and eczema in Chapter 3).

General questions

I have heard that people can develop allergies to certain substances and chemicals found in their place of work.

How commonly does this happen? Can these allergies affect all parts of the body?

In spite of extensive legislation, including the Health and Safety at Work Act of 1974, exposure to allergic sensitizers in the workplace is still very common. To give you some idea of the scale of the problem, approximately 900,000 working days a year are lost because of occupational dermatitis. Occupational asthma accounts for 2% of all adult asthma, with over 1,000 new cases occurring every year.

Occupational allergies most commonly cause allergic inflammation of the skin (dermatitis). Occupational asthma is the next most common form of workplace allergy, followed by inflammation of the nose (rhinitis), inflammation of the eye (conjunctivitis) and – but rarely – bowel allergies.

Do employers have any responsibility in the prevention of workplace allergies?

Yes. Employers have a legal duty to protect their employees from hazards in the workplace, and these include the development of allergic sensitization.

If you have developed an allergy to a substance used in your place of work, then the outlook is good and there is a reasonable chance that your symptoms will disappear – providing that the allergy is diagnosed early and from that point on you avoid the problem substance. If your allergy is more longstanding, avoidance of the cause will improve your symptoms, but they may not disappear completely. Because of this, all employers should aim to prevent the development of workplace allergies in the first place by identifying possible sensitizers, by assessing the level of risk to their employees from these sensitizers, and by protecting the workforce from these substances.

Your employer should also provide you with sufficient information and training so that you can identify potential risks to health, use control measures properly, and recognise even seemingly minor symptoms at an early stage. The Health and Safety Executive (address in Appendix 2) produces a large number of leaflets on these topics which you (and your employer!) might find useful.

Who is the best person to talk to if you think you have an allergy that is caused by your work?

If you work for a large organisation with an occupational health team, then you may be able to consult a nurse, works doctor or an employment medical advisor during your working hours. On the other hand, if you are one of only a handful of employees, then the first person you approach will probably be your GP. Any of these people should be able to help you in deciding whether or not your problem is connected with work, or to refer you for further tests or specialist advice.

However, your question could be interpreted another way – you may already know that you have an allergy caused by your work and be looking for someone to help you take action to protect you from further exposure to whatever is causing the problem. In a large company with a good health and safety record, a member of the occupational health team, a safety officer, or your manager or supervisor should be able to tell you what to do next: there may well be a set procedure for dealing with work-related health matters. In a small organisation, you will almost certainly need to talk directly to your employer. Unfortunately there are bad employers around as well as good ones. If you are concerned that you may get a negative reaction, and you are a member of a staff association, trade union, professional organisation or similar body, then you may want to approach them for advice before you do anything else. As a last resort, you could contact the Health and Safety Executive (address in Appendix 2).

Factory work

A year ago, at the age of 38, I developed asthma. This always seems to get better when I am on holiday from my job on an electrical factory production line, which I have been doing for the last 20 years. My doctor says that my asthma must be due to stress, and this is why it gets better when I am relaxing on holiday. I suspect that it might be

**something to do with my work, although why it should have
suddenly come on after so long, I don't know. How can I
sort out the cause of my asthma?**

You can become sensitized to a substance with which you have
worked without problems for many years. In your case it is likely
that rosin (a substance used in soldering, also called colophony)
is responsible for your asthma.

What makes me suspect that your asthma is due to your job is
the way it gets better when you are away from work. When
occupational asthma first develops, it often shows a pattern of
being worse during the week and better at weekends and during
holidays. As the asthma becomes more established, this pattern
may continue, or the asthma may become more chronic and
persist even during holidays. Occupational asthma does not tend
to show the seasonal variations which are so typical of other
forms of asthma. Although stress can certainly make asthma
worse, the pattern you describe strongly suggests an
occupational cause, which must be investigated.

Your next step should be to contact your works doctor or your
employment medical advisor, who will know how to proceed. It
is likely that you will be given a simple device called a peak flow
meter, which measures how hard you can blow air out from your
lungs (there is more information on this device and how to use it
in the sections on *Diagnosis and assessment* in Chapter 2 and
on *Peak expiratory flow testing* in Appendix 1). You will be
asked to measure your peak flow at two-hourly intervals
throughout the day, both on the days you spend at work and on
your days off. These readings should continue for at least two
weeks. If your asthma is due to an allergen in your workplace,
your peak flow recordings will show one of two distinctive
patterns. There may be a deterioration on each working day, with
a rapid recovery on leaving work. Alternatively, there may be a
progressive deterioration throughout the working week, with the
drop in your readings being greater at the end of the week than at
the beginning, and with recovery taking up to three days.

If you are shown to have occupational asthma, you must stop
working with the substance which has caused it. If you are

judged to have lost at least 14% of your lung function, you will be eligible for compensation. A good start would be for you to get hold of the Department of Social Security's leaflet NI 237 which is called *If you have asthma because of your work*, and then to arrange for your GP to refer you to your nearest allergy specialist.

I have recently developed asthma, caused by exposure to an antibiotic which is produced by the factory in which I work. I can't understand why I am the only one of all of my workmates to have developed this. Why is this?

There seems to be no obvious reason why one person develops an occupational allergy when another does not. Even people who smoke or who have a pre-existing health problem seem to be at no extra risk of this type of problem.

You have developed asthma because you have been exposed to a respiratory sensitizer, which is a substance known to act as an allergen in the production of allergy. Although you are the only one of your workmates to have developed such an allergy at present, it is possible that any one of them might develop a similar problem in the future. It is therefore essential that your employers take every possible step to eliminate the risk to their workforce caused by exposure to this antibiotic. This can be done by reducing the amount of antibiotic dust becoming airborne, by improving ventilation, by changing working techniques to limit the workforce's exposure, and by reducing the number of people who are exposed. Dust levels should be assessed regularly to check that these measures are effective. If these recommended measures do not reduce the dust to acceptable levels, then protective breathing equipment should be issued, but only as a last resort.

If you have any difficulty in getting your employer to take this problem seriously, please contact the Health and Safety Executive (address in Appendix 2) for advice.

I am in the process of applying for a job in a factory, and I have been asked to fill in an extensive health questionnaire. I have several minor health problems, including asthma, and I am concerned that I am going to be

discriminated against on the basis of health. Is this possible, and do I have to answer the questions?

It is becoming routine these days for employers to ask prospective employees about their health, even though there are no specified medical standards for most jobs. A good employer will want to give everyone a fair chance, and will not want to lose the opportunity of taking on a good employee because of unnecessary worries about health issues. Providing that you are able to do the job properly, and that you will not be a danger to yourself or to anyone else, then there is no reason why this employer should not take you on.

It sounds to me as if your asthma is irrelevant to your ability to work, assuming that your symptoms are well controlled. Even if there is a risk of becoming sensitized to certain allergens in this factory, you are not likely to be at significantly greater risk of sensitization than anyone else, unless your work is likely to involve platinum salts, enzyme detergents or animal proteins. It is only for these particular sensitizers that a pre-existing history of an allergic disorder such as asthma is likely to be grounds for exclusion from a particular job.

Unfortunately your worries about discrimination are not without foundation. As things stand at present, if you are asked about your health on an application form or at an interview and you do not disclose the full facts, then at any time in the future you can be dismissed for not revealing the information. At the moment there is no legal protection for applicants refused a job on account of their health (even if you could prove that that was the real reason), and almost none for employees dismissed because of their health record. You might decide that you want to take the risk and keep quiet about your medical history, but a more sensible option would be to phrase your answers to the questionnaire as positively as possible, and in a way that convinces your potential employer that your asthma will not affect your ability to do the job.

In the past I developed a serious dermatitis on my hands which proved to be due to a latex allergy. Does this mean

**that I am prone to developing chemical allergies, and what
can I do to avoid problems in the future?**

As you have developed one chemical sensitivity, it is possible that
you could develop others. As well as making sure you avoid
contact with latex, there are certain things that you can do to
reduce the chances of contact dermatitis in the future.

- Avoid materials that carry a manufacturer's skin hazard
  warning.
- Avoid rough or abrasive hand work.
- Avoid getting your hands excessively wet.
- Always wash your hands properly after handling any potential
  irritant.
- Protect your hands when working with solvents, glues, grease
  or oil, and corrosive chemicals.
- Avoid extremes of temperature and humidity.
- At work use any form of protection offered including barrier
  creams, after-wash creams, gloves (but NOT latex ones!) and
  washing facilities.
- Do not use solvents to remove substances from your hands, as
  the solvents themselves can cause dermatitis.

**I went to my doctor recently for help and advice about
some symptoms that I had put down to hayfever. I get an
itchy and runny nose, red sore runny eyes, and feel a bit
tight in my chest. He pointed out that hayfever doesn't
very often come on at my age (I am 45), nor does it often
start in the winter. He went on to ask me about my job: I
work in a textiles factory using a dyeing process. Could
these dyes really be causing my problems, and might I now
lose my job?**

It sounds as if you have an excellent doctor! He is right: although
the symptoms of hayfever can start at any age and can occur at
any time of year, your symptoms do sound rather unusual, and I
think it is perfectly possible that they are being caused by an
allergic reaction to the dyestuffs you use at work. Modern dyes
(particularly a group called the reactive dyes) commonly cause
allergy, which not only affects the skin and the lungs, but also the

nose and the eyes. Your GP will probably refer you to a specialist allergy clinic where you can be tested for such an allergy. Not only will they perform skin prick testing, but there is also a blood test available called RAST which looks for specific antibodies to these dyes (these tests are described in Appendix 1).

If you turn out to be allergic to the dyes used at work, it is essential that you avoid further exposure. You should tell your charge hand, foreman, safety officer, union safety representative or works manager about your allergy as soon as possible. Your employer and the supplier of the dyes are required by law to take precautions for your health and safety. They must assess any risk to your health, prevent or control your exposure, and keep a check on any effects the dyes may have on your health. You on your part are required to make full and proper use of any equipment and facilities provided by your employer, to take reasonable care for your own health and safety, and to co-operate with your employer on matters of health and safety. You should keep all items of protective clothing and equipment separate from your outer clothing; you should wash your hands, arms and face thoroughly with soap and water (or have a shower) before going home; and you should never use organic solvents to clean dye stains from your skin. If your problems persist despite these precautions, then your employer should move you to a job in which you will not be exposed to these dyes.

Working outdoors

My 18-year-old son has just taken up a job as a trainee gardener. Since starting work he has developed very sore and itchy hands, with blistering at times. He is very reluctant to tell his employer or to go to our doctor as he loves the job and would hate to lose it. Is this likely to be an allergy, and what is likely to be causing it?

It does sound as if his problem is allergic in nature. A wide range of plants can start off an allergic process and cause contact dermatitis (the medical name for your son's skin problems).

Among those commonly encountered in this country and well-known to cause skin problems are:

- Alstroemeria;
- Chrysanthemums and various other members of the daisy family;
- Daphne (some species only);
- Ivics;
- Leyland cypress;
- Primula obconica;
- Schefflera; and
- bulbs such as tulips, lilies, hyacinths and narcissus.

A form of skin testing called patch testing (described in Appendix 1) may well be able to identify the culprit. If he is only allergic to one or two plants, it might be possible for him to avoid these completely. If not, he could make sure he always wear gloves whenever he has to handle them. Only if his symptoms persist despite these measures will he have to reassess whether or not this is the right job for him.

My husband is a forestry worker and (although he won't admit it) his asthma was very much worse in autumn and early winter last year. He had some really bad attacks, and slept extremely badly. He was very much better during the Christmas holiday, when we mostly stayed at home. Was this coincidence, or could there be something about his job that makes his asthma worse?

Almost certainly the triggers for your husband's asthma last autumn were the spores produced by moulds and fungi, which grow particularly well in the dark damp conditions of a forest. I would advise him to go to see his doctor, who will prescribe treatment with adequate levels of preventative (anti-inflammatory) medications to keep his asthma under control. Your GP may also give your husband a peak flow meter so that he can keep a record of his lung function on a day to day basis. Your husband may require extra medication during the mould spore season, which starts in September. His peak flow recordings will be useful in showing what level of treatment he requires.

There is more information on peak flow recordings in the sections on *Diagnosis and assessment* in Chapter 2 and on *Peak expiratory flow testing* in Appendix 1, and on preventative treatment for asthma in the section on *Treatment* in Chapter 2.

Office work

I am a secretary, and work on a computer with a VDU screen for up to eight hours a day. I have terrible problems with my eyes: they always feel tired and dry and itchy, and now my face is also red and itchy. I am sure the VDU is the cause, but my boss disagrees. Who is right?

Visual display units (VDUs) have been in use for a long time, and are now virtually everywhere. Like you, some people find that they develop sore eyes when working long hours with these screens. This is because people blink less when staring at a VDU screen than they normally do. Because of this, tears (the eye's natural lubricant) are less well distributed over the eye, which therefore becomes slightly dry and irritated. You can reduce the problem by making sure that you have frequent breaks from looking at your screen. The VDU should be positioned carefully so as not to be against a bright light or window, and so as not to reflect bright lights in the screen. A filter fitted over your VDU screen will also help to reduce glare.

There have been a number of reports of redness and itching of the face in VDU workers. This might be caused by the combination of a dry atmosphere in the workplace and increased static electricity near the VDU. Try using a simple emollient cream such as E45 (available from most chemists) and, if the condition does not improve, arrange to see your doctor.

Finally, some people do worry that they are being affected by radiation from VDUs, but this is very unlikely to be the cause of any problems. VDUs do give off a small amount of radiation, but this is less than the amount given off by the average human body, which is itself slightly radioactive.

I always feel unwell at work, but feel much better at weekends. Several of my colleagues in the office find the same. We think that our building has sick building syndrome. What causes this?

A few years ago there were many reports of supposed sick building syndrome, and a number of studies have been carried out to investigate this phenomenon. It does appear that certain buildings can make the people working in them feel unwell, but no one is sure why this happens. One of the suggested causes was a high concentration of the house dust mite. However, allergy to the house dust mite generally causes clear-cut allergic symptoms such as asthma, rhinitis or eczema, whereas your symptoms sound rather more generalised.

Air-conditioning (which makes the air very dry) or overheating (due to lack of natural ventilation) could both be responsible for making you feel generally off-colour. You could try getting outside for a walk and some fresh air as often as you reasonably can during the day, and see if this helps solve your problem. And have you considered whether you are happy at work, or if you dislike your job for some reason? Feeling negative about your work, which fills a considerable proportion of your waking hours, could add to your feeling unwell during the week.

I would advise you to see your doctor who will give you a general checkup and who will also arrange for allergy testing if this seems to be appropriate.

Other occupations

I have developed bad eczema on my hands since becoming an assistant chef. This seems to be because of an allergy to the foodstuffs that I handle. Is this possible? I have also been told that I must stay off work until my hands recover, because I am putting customers at risk of food poisoning. How can this be?

It is most likely that your problem is not in fact eczema, but a form of contact dermatitis, which can be caused by a wide range of foodstuffs. People working in catering are particularly at risk as their hands are often wet and they frequently suffer small cuts: both these factors allow allergens to penetrate the skin.

I would recommend that you see your doctor urgently and ask for a referral to a dermatologist (a doctor who specialises in treatment of the skin and its problems), as you cannot return to work until the problem is cleared up. The specialist should be able to identify which foodstuffs are causing the problem, either by patch testing or by using RAST (both these tests are described in Appendix 1). Once the cause of your dermatitis has been identified, you might be able to avoid contact with it – wearing plastic gloves may help. However, if the problem continues, you might unfortunately have to consider changing your career, as your employer is perfectly correct: severe contact dermatitis on the hands can become infected with organisms which, if passed on to the food, can cause food poisoning.

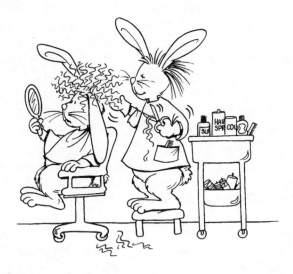

I am a hairdressing trainee, and recently I developed a nasty inflammation on my hands. My boss suggested I started wearing gloves, but since then my hands have got very much worse, and I now can't work. What is causing this awful irritation, and what can I do?

I suspect that the initial soreness and inflammation of your hands was due to irritation from the chemicals used in hairdressing. To combat this you started wearing gloves, which probably contained latex. I think you may now have developed a latex allergy, and the recent more severe dermatitis you are experiencing is from the gloves, rather than from the hairdressing chemicals.

There are a number of things you can try which might improve the condition of your hands.

* Keep your hands clean and dry whenever possible.
* Ask your employer for plastic (latex-free) gloves, which you should wear only when absolutely necessary, in order to avoid getting chemicals onto your skin.
* Be very careful with anything which might scratch or cut your hands.
* Ask your doctor to arrange for you to be tested for allergy to latex as well as to the common hairdressing chemicals.

If you prove to be allergic to latex but not to any of the hairdressing chemicals, then I can see no reason why you can't continue in your present job (making sure that you always use latex-free plastic gloves when you need to protect your hands). If, however, you prove to be allergic to any of the dyeing or perming solutions, then you might have to rethink your choice of career.

I work in a garage. A month or two ago I developed really sore hands, and since then have been making sure that I remove as much of the oil and grease from my hands at the end of the day as possible by using a solvent. Despite that, my hands seem to be getting worse and worse. What can I do?

The first thing you should do is to stop using the solvent! Although this may appear to remove the oil and grease from your hands, it actually allows a greater amount of these substances to penetrate your skin, and can itself cause allergies.

Your problem sounds like a form of contact dermatitis caused by one of the chemicals with which your hands come into contact. From now on, you should try to protect your hands from all oil, grease, lubricants and fuel oils, either by wearing gloves or by using a suitable barrier cream (your employer should be able to provide this for you) which should be put on at the beginning of the day when your skin is completely clean. At the end of the day, clean your hands with a detergent-based rather than a solvent-based preparation. If your problem persists despite these efforts, I suggest that you ask your doctor to refer you to a dermatologist for allergy testing.

My 16-year-old daughter has started a Saturday job in a pet shop. She loves animals and hopes to pursue a career as a veterinary nurse. The problem is that her eczema, which she has had off and on since infancy, has got dramatically worse, and I think sometimes I can hear her wheezing. She says everything is fine and refuses to go to the doctor but I am very worried about her. Could her Saturday job be responsible? By the way, we don't have any pets at home because my husband is allergic to both cats and dogs.

I think your daughter is almost certainly allergic to one or more of the animals that she cares for at work. As she loves animals, she probably spends as much time with them as possible, stroking and petting them and so getting large doses of allergen onto her skin and into her lungs in the process.

The first thing to do is to advise your daughter not to pick up or pet any of the animals at work. I would recommend that she sees your doctor as soon as possible to ask if she can be skin tested for common animal allergens such as cat, dog, guinea-pig and horse. Your GP will also prescribe appropriate treatment for her eczema, and will ask her to keep regular recordings of her lung function to see whether or not she is developing asthma (if so, she may require treatment for this as well). This is a simple test, which is done at home using a portable peak flow meter and is explained further in the sections on *Diagnosis and assessment* in Chapter 2 and on *Peak expiratory flow testing* in Appendix 1.

Once her symptoms are under control and you have the results of the allergy tests, then you, your doctor and your daughter can discuss together whether she should give up her Saturday job, and whether she would be wise to rethink her future career.

I was made redundant last year, and have recently set myself up as a self-employed painter and decorator. I have always been in good health up until now, but over the past few months I have noticed that my chest often feels very tight and I have difficulty breathing when I am at work. Could I be reacting to one of the paints I use, and if so, how do I find out which one?

Paints are made from a wide range of chemical substances including pigments, solvents, dryers and extenders. Some of these can act as irritants, and some of them can also be responsible for causing an allergy – as sounds likely in your case.

It may prove very difficult to find out which paint is causing your allergy, but you may find the following pieces of advice helpful.

- Use water-based paints wherever possible.
- Make sure the room in which you are working is as well-ventilated as possible.
- Always replace the lids on containers to prevent the release of fumes and vapours into the atmosphere.
- Keep your work area as dust-free as possible.
- Never eat, drink or smoke while painting.
- Take care when cleaning your brushes and other equipment so as not to spray fine particles into the air.
- Wash your hands and take off your protective clothing before going home.
- Consider using a respirator fitted with an appropriate filter.

If your symptoms persist, you should ask your GP to refer you to a specialist allergy clinic where they might be able to identify the substance causing your allergy. You might then be able to avoid using paints or solvents containing this particular chemical.

8
Living with allergies

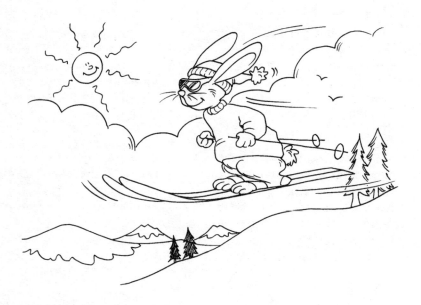

Introduction

This chapter deals with some of the very practical questions about everyday matters which are frequently asked by people with allergies of all types. It covers a broad sweep of topics, but concentrates on those situations when having an allergy can pose particular problems. Going on holiday, going to school and being admitted to hospital (perhaps for an operation totally unconnected with your allergy, perhaps because you are having a baby) will all involve you in meeting new experiences. Certain aspects of your life will be outside your control, for example where you sleep and what you are offered to eat. These changes can cause anxiety and, as we all know, anxiety in itself can make allergies worse. I hope that the information given here – combined with a bit of forward planning – will help you to cope better with these events And, in the case of holidays, to enjoy them!

Holidays and travel

I have never had a holiday abroad as I am too frightened that my asthma will get worse and that something awful will happen. Am I being unnecessarily cautious?

Obviously you shouldn't go abroad on holiday unless you think you would enjoy it, but I do think you are probably being a little over-cautious in not allowing yourself to try a foreign holiday at all. You are particularly concerned about your asthma, but people with other allergies (or other medical conditions entirely) have worries about foreign travel which are very similar to yours. If you can work out exactly what it is about going abroad that troubles you, then you can plan how to avoid that problem or what to do if it occurs.

- If it is the thought of language problems that worries you – that you might not be able to make yourself understood to people in your holiday resort or to health care professionals – then why not consider a holiday in an English-speaking country?
- If it is the thought of flying that worries you, why not travel to continental Europe by sea or via the Channel Tunnel?
- If you are concerned about the standard of medical care abroad, why not choose a country with a modern and efficient health service? You may feel better when you remember that asthma and other allergies are common in many countries, so that wherever you are (providing that you are not too far off the beaten track), it is likely that the doctors are highly experienced in dealing with these conditions.

There are sensible precautions that you can take to try and ensure your holiday is as trouble-free as possible as far as your health and its care is concerned, and these are discussed in the following answers in this section. I hope you are reassured that with sufficient advanced planning it is possible for people with allergies to travel safely and enjoyably anywhere they wish to go, and that you now have the confidence to try a holiday abroad. Perhaps a good way to start would be with a short holiday somewhere not too far afield, with a tour operator who will provide you with the services of an English-speaking representative.

Before I leave to go on holiday I try to make sure I have enough medication to last whilst I'm away, but are there any other precautions I should take?

There are, and forward planning is well worth the effort as it will help to make sure that your holiday is a success. You may find some or all of the following points helpful.

- Choose the holiday destination which is the least likely to trigger your particular allergy. There is no best place to go, but from your past experience you may know of places to avoid.
- Contact your holiday company well in advance to ask for any specific requirements, such as feather-free bedding or a special diet. Ask them to confirm in writing that they will be able to meet your special needs, and take their letter with you when you go in case of any administrative slip-ups on their part.
- Make sure that your symptoms are as well controlled as possible before you go on holiday. If you are at all concerned, visit your GP in plenty of time so that any necessary adjustments can be made to your treatment.
- Ask your GP to provide you with a written plan explaining what you should do if your allergy gets worse while you are away. For example, if you have asthma, your doctor may prescribe a course of oral steroid tablets for you to take should you need them.
- Arrange adequate medical insurance to cover you while you are away, and get good advice on how much cover you may need (health care costs vary considerably in different parts of

the world). Remember to give details of your allergy on the insurance application form – if you do not mention it, it will not be covered.

- Medical attention is officially free in all European Union countries provided that you have completed form E111 (which you can get from a Post Office) before you leave home. You should remember to do this even if you are only going across the Channel for a day's shopping or a short break.
- Make sure that you carry supplies of all your medications in your hand luggage so that they are readily accessible. And carry a back-up supply in a separate bag, in case one bag is lost or stolen.
- When you arrive at your destination, find out where the nearest telephone is, how to call for a doctor and an ambulance, and the whereabouts of the nearest hospital casualty (accident & emergency) department.
- Make sure your travelling companions know about your allergy and how to help you should you have an acute problem.
- Take this book with you if you have space in your luggage! It will be a source of information for both you and your companions. Another publication you may find useful is the *Traveller's Guide to Health* which is produced by the Department of Health (details of how to obtain a copy are in Appendix 3).

Can I get supplies of my usual medication in other countries if I need to for any reason, say if all my luggage is stolen?

As you do not say what treatment you are taking or for which allergy, I can only answer your question in general terms.

- Most of the commonly-prescribed allergy treatments are available in other economically-developed countries, but may be more difficult to obtain in more exotic or remote holiday destinations.
- Recently-developed drugs may only be available in a limited number of countries.
- The formulation, strength and brand name of your usual

treatment may be different in another country. All drugs have two names: a generic name and a brand (or trade) name. The generic name is the true or scientific name of the drug, given to it when it is first developed, and that name normally remains the same wherever you are in the world. The brand name is the name given to the drug by the manufacturer, and that name can vary from country to country, or from manufacturer to manufacturer if it is made by more than one pharmaceutical company.

The medical information departments of the major pharmaceutical companies will be able to tell you which of their products are available in which countries and under what names. I suggest that you check with the company making your particular treatment before you travel, and take a note of the details with you, including the generic name of your medication.

I worry that my medication might be confiscated when I go through customs. Could this happen, and if so, what should I do?

If you are travelling to Western Europe, North America, Australia or New Zealand, then there should be no problems about your medication, as it is unlikely that it will be confiscated. Allergies are common and well recognised in these parts of the world – for example, as many as 10% of travellers might be carrying asthma inhalers – so customs officers are used to seeing people who need to keep their routine medication with them.

If you are travelling further afield, then it might be wise to carry a letter from your doctor explaining what your medication is for, why you must carry it, and confirming that it has been prescribed for your personal use. Such a letter will not guarantee that your medication will not be confiscated by customs, but it might prove useful if you have any difficulties. You might also find it worthwhile to contact the embassies of the countries you are visiting to ask for their advice before you leave.

I am only going away for a short time. Would it be all right to stop my treatment while I am away?

No it would not be all right! Even if you are only away for a short period of time, you must continue to take your prescribed treatment or your allergy could get worse and spoil your holiday. For example, if you have asthma and you stop taking your preventer inhaler regularly, then you run the risk of precipitating a general worsening of your asthma and even of provoking a severe asthma attack. As well as using your preventer inhaler regularly, you should also always carry your reliever inhaler with you. It could be very dangerous for you not to have the means of treating your asthma symptoms should they occur while you are on holiday.

I have asthma. Is it safe for me to fly?

Yes. Modern aeroplanes are pressurised so that conditions inside them are almost the same as on the ground. Make sure when you book your seat that you are as far away as possible from the smoking section, or, even better, fly with an airline which bans smoking altogether. If you might need to use a nebuliser on board, warn the airline when you book your seat. They may be able to provide you with a nebuliser, or will be able to arrange for you to use your own. Make sure that you take all your medications on board with you, as although most airlines carry a small supply of medications, these might not be your usual ones. Try to plan your journey carefully so that you avoid situations which might make you anxious or upset, as these emotions might bring on your asthma.

I have been offered a promotion at work, and my new job would involve a lot of travelling, particularly to America. Is this a good idea, as I suffer from both asthma and hayfever?

Providing that you are conscientious about taking your preventer treatments for your asthma (remembering to allow for the differences in time zones), and follow the other advice for trouble-free travelling given in this section, then there is no reason why you should not be able to travel frequently without too many problems.

Are there any holiday activities that I should avoid because of my asthma?

The only one I can think of is scuba diving. This can be dangerous because of the risk of having an acute attack under water, and because of the problems associated with breathing compressed air. However, other activities which are particularly exhilarating (such as parachuting), or which involve moving in restricted spaces (such as potholing) should probably also be regarded with caution. Otherwise, providing that your asthma is well controlled, and you have your reliever inhaler with you, you should be able to participate in almost all holiday activities.

Can I take my nebuliser abroad?

Assuming that the voltage of the power supply in the country you are visiting is similar to that in the United Kingdom (240 volts) then all you will need to be able to use your nebuliser is an adapter for the plug. The compressors of some modern nebulisers have an integral battery so they can be used independently of the mains for a while, but as these batteries have only a limited life, even these will need a power supply at some stage for recharging them.

If the voltage is different (as in the United States) you will not be able to use your nebuliser unless it has a dual voltage facility.

I am allergic to peanuts. How can I be sure that I'm not given food with peanuts in whilst I'm on holiday ?

The safest way to ensure that you do not inadvertently eat food containing peanuts is to prepare all of your food yourself. However, a self-catering holiday is not everybody's idea of a perfect break!

If you want to eat commercially prepared meals, then it is essential that you are able to explain to the people serving and cooking your food that you are unable to eat peanuts. If you are not fluent in the language of the country you are visiting, then it might help to take a pre-prepared card with you, giving the necessary details in the appropriate language, which you could then show whenever you needed to. You may need help in preparing the card (it is obviously important that it is correct) –

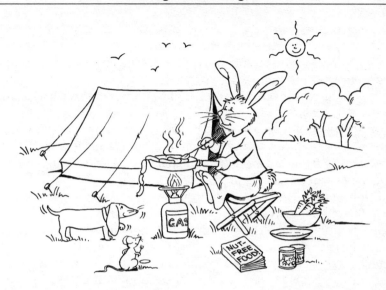

perhaps a local language teacher could help, or you could contact the Institute of Translation and Interpreting (address in Appendix 2). The British Allergy Foundation and the Anaphylaxis Campaign (again the addresses are in Appendix 2) produce a series of pre-prepared cards in various languages, and you might find one of these is exactly what you need.

Accidents can still happen, so you must carry your treatment with you at all times, in the form of either an Epipen or an Anapen. Make sure that your adrenaline preparation has not reached its expiry date, and that both you and your travelling companions know how to administer it. You will find more information about adrenaline in the section on **Emergency treatment** in Chapter 6.

I am very allergic to insect bites, and I'm dreading my holiday because I always seem to get bitten to death! Is there anything I can do to put the insects off me? They never seem to bite my husband!

Yes, there are a number of things that you can try to prevent being bitten by insects.

- Cover as much of your body as possible when spending time out of doors, especially in the evening.
- If possible, avoid being out of doors in the evening, when insects are much more active.
- Wear light-coloured clothing. Bright colours and dark clothing attract insects.
- Avoid perfume and scented skin creams, deodorants, cosmetics, hair spray, etc. The smell attracts insects.
- Stay away from areas such as gardens, rubbish bins, and picnic grounds where insects are likely to be found.
- If you are on a self-catering holiday, keep kitchen areas and rubbish bins clean and free from food scraps.
- Before going out of doors, use a good quality insect repellent on all exposed skin surfaces, avoiding your lips and eyes. You may find that an insect repellent bought locally is more effective against that country's insect population.
- There is some evidence that certain insects (particularly mosquitoes) dislike the taste and smell of vitamin B_1 (thiamine). Try taking 100 mg of vitamin B_1 once a day, starting two weeks before you go away and continuing throughout your holiday.

School

My 4-year-old daughter, who has asthma, is about to start school. What information should I give her teachers?

The school will probably already be familiar with the problems that asthma can cause because as many as one in eight children of this age have asthma. However, it would still be sensible to provide your daughter's teacher with some written details, which should include the following information.

- The medications your daughter routinely needs to take at school, for example a midday dose of her preventer inhaler.
- Details of any medications she takes before exercise.
- A treatment plan of exactly what to do should her asthma suddenly get worse.

- Telephone numbers where you, your partner or another responsible relative can be contacted at all times.
- The telephone number of your daughter's doctor.
- Information about things known to trigger your daughter's asthma, for example pets, exercise and excitement.

You may find it useful to give the school some more general information about asthma. The National Asthma Campaign and the National Asthma and Respiratory Training Centre (addresses in Appendix 2) both produce excellent information packs for schools.

Every school should now have its own asthma policy, which will probably be based on one suggested by the National Asthma Campaign. The Department for Education and Employment is also producing guidelines for the management of asthma in schools. With all this information available, your daughter's teachers should feel well equipped to cope with her asthma.

I have three children and they all have allergies, although only one of them has asthma. I assume the sort of information I give their teachers will be much the same for all of them, but do schools know as much about other allergies as they do about asthma?

You are perfectly correct, the information that teachers need is much the same, whatever a child's allergy. You could use the list in the previous answer as a starting point, simply adapting it where necessary to cover each child's particular needs. However, although all schools should now have an asthma policy, the same is not true of other allergic problems, so they will probably appreciate extra information about your children's particular allergies. As well as specific instructions about each of your children, why not offer the school some of the leaflets produced by the British Allergy Foundation (address in Appendix 2), or even suggest that the pupils do a project on the subject of allergy?

My son's school won't let him carry his own asthma inhalers, but makes him go to the school secretary each time he needs to use them. He often doesn't bother. Will this harm him?

It is important that your son takes his asthma medication as prescribed by your doctor. If he needs to take his preventer inhaler at midday then yes, it could be harmful for him to miss this dose, as the control of his asthma is likely to suffer. It is just as worrying if he is not taking his reliever inhaler whenever he needs it. Ideally this inhaler should be kept with him all the time, so that he has immediate access to it.

Unfortunately, many schools have a policy that all medications needed by children should be locked away. This is usually done from the best of motives – they may be worried that a child will lose their medication, or that it will be stolen, or misused by another child in the class. However, in the case of asthma this is potentially dangerous, and the Department of Health has recommended that all children should have immediate access to their inhalers. This recommendation will soon be included in the *Children's Charter* (details of how to obtain a copy are in Appendix 3).

I suggest that you discuss all this with your son's teachers and try to persuade them to alter their current policy. You could also ask your doctor to write to the school, explaining why it is best that your son has immediate access to his inhalers at all times. You may be able to come to a compromise with the school: perhaps they could keep spare inhalers for your son in case he forgets or loses one. You will also need to persuade your son of the importance of taking his inhalers as prescribed, even if it is a little inconvenient for him (I realise that this is easier said than done).

I have heard that some children have been turned away from nursery schools and playgroups because the staff are not prepared to be responsible for adrenaline injections. Is this true? And what about when the children are older – does this apply to infant and junior schools as well?

Unfortunately you are right. Some private nurseries and playgroups have refused entry to children with severe allergies because, for various reasons, the staff were not prepared to take responsibility for the children's emergency treatment. I think this is very sad, as not only does it stigmatise the affected children, but also because the staff have missed out on an opportunity to become better informed about allergic problems. However, if these were private establishments, they will have been acting entirely within their rights.

The situation is different for children in state schools. All children, including those with medical needs, have a right to a full education, and the teachers in these schools should be prepared, within reason, to take responsibility for children's medical needs whilst they are in school. In October 1996 the Department for Education and Employment and the Department of Health jointly issued guidelines on supporting pupils with medical needs in school. These guidelines included details of the responsibilities of education staff, advice on drawing up school policies, and brief information on some medical conditions. Copies can be obtained free from the Department for Education and Employment (address in Appendix 2.).

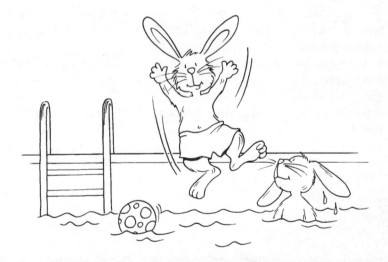

My son has eczema, which at times can be quite severe. I am very concerned as next term his class are to have some intensive swimming instruction. I want him to be able to take part in this, so is there anything I can do to improve his skin beforehand? And is there anything I should do to

**protect his skin from the effect of the chemicals in the
water?**

Eczema can pose a number of problems for children when they
start to go swimming. Firstly, children can be very shy about the
appearance of their skin, often to the extent that they do not want
to join in, and secondly, as you rightly say, there is the concern
that the chemicals in the swimming pool water may make eczema
worse.

There are indeed steps you can take to try and make the
condition of your son's skin better before the start of next term.

- You could check with your doctor that the skin preparations
  you are using are the best ones for your son.
- You should be careful to apply his different skin creams as
  frequently as you are meant to – it is easy to forget!
- Make sure that he has at least one bath a day with plenty of
  dispersible emollient in the water.
- If you know that there are factors which make his eczema
  worse, such as certain foods, then try to avoid these over the
  next month or so.
- Make sure that your son wears natural fibres such as cotton
  next to his skin, and avoid clothes made from wool, as these
  can be very irritating.
- If you know that your son is allergic to the house dust mite, you
  might consider buying him a full set of anti-allergy bedding
  covers.

With any luck, if you follow these pieces of advice your son's skin
will be in good condition by the time his swimming course starts.
However, he will also need to take special care of his skin after
each swimming session.

- He must have a shower after swimming and he should take his
  soap substitute with him and use it (normal soap can be very
  drying).
- He should, if possible, moisturise his skin with his normal
  emollient (moisturising and softening cream) after his shower,
  before putting on his clothes.

You may need to enlist his teachers' support, as often the children are rushed to and from the pool and are not given enough time for a shower. Once the teachers appreciate how important this is, I am sure they will agree to help.

My daughter has various food allergies and I am worried about how she will cope with meals when she starts school. What can I do to stop her eating the foods that upset her so badly?

The first solution I can offer is to suggest that you provide your daughter with a packed lunch. However, that might not solve the problem, as children often share one another's lunches and you will not be able to be certain that she eats her own and not someone else's food. Would one of the teachers be prepared to supervise your daughter while she is eating her meal?

Alternatively, you could arrange for your daughter to have school meals, but again you would need to ask whether a teacher or dining room supervisor could help her to select appropriate foods. You would need to explain to the member of staff exactly what your daughter is and is not allowed to eat.

This is a problem that should improve with time. As your daughter gets older, it will be increasingly easy for her to understand that there are certain foods she should not eat, and she is also likely to grow out of some of her food allergies.

If she has a serious allergy to one or more foods, it is important that both she and the staff (dining room staff as well as teachers) know what to do should she eat the wrong food by mistake.

Is it all right to send my son to school when his skin is bad or when he is wheezy? He has both asthma and eczema.

It depends how bad his skin is, and how severe his wheezing.

Taking the wheezing first, if he is only slightly wheezy, or is getting over a cold but is well in himself, it should be perfectly safe to send him to school. Similarly, if his chest is a little wheezy because he is upset (perhaps for some reason he doesn't want to go to school), then providing that you can make sure he has access to his reliever inhaler throughout the school day, he should again be able to go to school. If, however, your son is just developing an attack of asthma, or is wheezy enough for it to interfere with normal everyday tasks, then it would be safer to keep him at home until the attack is under control. If you do send him to school, make sure the teachers are able to contact you should his asthma get worse.

If your son's eczema is particularly severe, he may not want to go to school as he may well suffer from teasing or unkind remarks from the other children. He may also feel under the weather because he is not sleeping well. If so, you might want to keep him at home for a few days until his skin has improved. Do arrange to see your son's GP if this happens a lot, as the doctor may be able to make useful changes to your son's treatment and advise you on whether there is anything else you can do, such as using anti-allergy bedding covers (discussed in the section on *House dust mite* in Chapter 9). If your son's eczema is relatively mild, there is no reason why he cannot go to school, although it would be helpful if he could take a tube of his emollient (moisturising and softening cream) with him to use if his skin is particularly itchy.

My daughter is being bullied. Could this be making her eczema worse?

Yes, the upset that bullying causes could be making her eczema worse. Stress is often a factor which is responsible for making allergic problems more severe. In your daughter's case it is affecting her eczema, but emotion can also be a strong trigger for asthma, and this type of emotional upset can be responsible for a deterioration in the control of a child's asthma.

I hope you find that once this problem has been tackled, her eczema is less troublesome.

Will my daughter's school make allowances for her hayfever when they mark her GCSEs, as the exams are at the time of year that her symptoms are at their very worst?

Many GCSE syllabuses contain a major in-course continuous assessment component, and so the examinations contribute less weight to the final result than they once did. However, they are still important and there are several steps you can take to ensure that your daughter's hayfever interferes with her exam performance as little as possible.

She should go to see her doctor well before the hayfever season commences, and start taking her recommended treatment before her symptoms appear. This will be much more effective than waiting until after her symptoms have begun. She may need to use a nasal spray as well as taking an antihistamine, and if her eyes are affected, then she may need eye drops as well (there is more information about all these medications in the section on *Treatment* in Chapter 4).

I hope that treatment along these lines will make sure that her symptoms are minimised. However, it would also be sensible to find out what should happen if her hayfever does affect her badly during her exams, especially as policy varies between examination boards. A letter from her doctor explaining her situation might be needed, for example, or her teacher might need to appeal to the board on her behalf. Have you considered asking her school to contact the relevant board well in advance of her exams to find out exactly what their attitude would be?

Is it safe for my son, who has asthma, to go on school trips, especially ones which involve overnight stays away from home? I do so want him to lead a normal life, but worry that he might have an attack and no one would know what to do.

It is understandable that you worry about your son. However, it is unlikely that he will be the only child with asthma on the school trip. Asthma is now so common among children that most teachers are very well informed about how to avoid attacks and also how to treat them if they do occur.

To be on the safe side, make sure your son's teachers know that he has asthma and give them written information about his treatment. This should include information on what to do if he does have an attack. You might also like to provide them with some general information about asthma which you could obtain from either the National Asthma Campaign or the National Asthma and Respiratory Training Centre (addresses in Appendix 2).

My daughter has severe asthma, and is losing a lot of schooling. Should she go to a special school?

Children with asthma should be encouraged to lead as normal a life as possible, and it is rarely necessary for them to attend special schools. However, if your daughter has asthma which is severe enough to interfere with her education, then it is important that you know how to make sure that she gets the most out of school and does not have to miss too many lessons.

The first thing to do is to check that her treatment is as effective as possible. Arrange to see your GP to discuss both her medication and her inhaler technique – it may be that something as simple as a change of inhaler will help improve the control of her asthma (there is more information about the different types of inhaler in the section on *Treatment* in Chapter 2).

Next I would suggest you make an appointment to see your daughter's form (class) teacher or head teacher to make sure that the school has an acceptable asthma policy. This should include a commitment to immediate access to reliever inhalers, staff training on asthma trigger factors, and a plan of action on how to deal with any acute attacks of asthma. If the school does not have such a policy, suggest that they send off for a schools information pack from the National Asthma Campaign or the National Asthma and Respiratory Training Centre (addresses in Appendix 2). They should also have a copy of *Supporting pupils with medical needs in schools*, which is published by the Department for Education and Employment.

If none of this works and your daughter continues to miss a lot of school, then you should contact your local education authority, who will have a person responsible for children with special educational needs. Having special educational needs is not related to your daughter's intelligence, but is a reflection of her academic, social and physical needs. It can be a very positive step to be identified as having these special needs, as then something can be done to help.

Every school has a special educational needs co-ordinator, who can arrange an individual learning programme for your daughter, talk to your doctor about ways to help her, and show you how you can give her further support. Her progress will be monitored regularly. If she needs even more help, then she will be given a detailed assessment which may, if her school problems are severe, lead to a formal statement of special educational needs. The statement sometimes leads to a recommendation for a special school placement, or it may recommend providing extra support to allow your daughter to remain in her current school. The process of obtaining a statement can take some time and it may require some persistence on your part, so you may want to start finding out about it now. The Department for Education and Employment publishes a booklet called *Special Educational Needs – A Guide for Parents* which outlines the procedures and explains the jargon used: details of how to obtain a copy are in Appendix 3.

Going into hospital

Is it safe for someone with asthma like me to have a general anaesthetic?

Provided that your asthma is under good control, it is almost as safe for you to have a general anaesthetic as any other person. It is important that you continue to take your regular preventer treatment in the month before your operation, and it would be sensible to monitor your asthma using a peak flow meter to ensure that your control is as good as possible (the use of peak flow meters is discussed in the sections on *Diagnosis and assessment* in Chapter 2 and on *Peak expiratory flow testing* in Appendix 1). If your peak flows show that your asthma control is not at its best, see your GP as soon as possible, so that your treatment can be adjusted.

It is very important that you tell your anaesthetist that you have asthma. As well as being a highly trained specialist in giving anaesthetics, an anaesthetist is a fully qualified doctor who will be able to ensure that your treatment continues right up to the time of your operation. The anaesthetist will probably suggest that you receive an extra dose of your reliever treatment with your premedication.

If your asthma is particularly severe, your anaesthetist might feel that it is better for you to have your operation performed under local anaesthetic. This is quite common these days, and can be used in a wide range of surgical procedures.

I have been told that you are not allowed to have a general anaesthetic while you have a cold. I am worried that I won't be able to have my operation because my hayfever is like a cold but all the year round. What should I do?

If you are having a routine operation, it is true that an anaesthetist would probably prefer you to be in perfect health before giving you an anaesthetic, and not to have a cold. It is not the blocked nose that the anaesthetist is concerned about, but the effects of the cold virus on the rest of your body. Your hayfever should not pose a problem. Just explain that it is hayfever and not a cold.

It sounds to me though as if your hayfever could be better treated. You may need to use a nasal spray as well as taking an antihistamine: this combination should be able to get rid of most of your symptoms. There is more information about these medications in the section on *Treatment* in Chapter 4.

Whilst I'm in hospital for my operation, will I be allowed to use my inhalers whenever I need to?

The ward nurses would probably prefer that you give them your preventer inhaler for safe keeping. It will then be prescribed for you on your treatment sheet, so you will still be able to use it according to your usual regime – it will be given to you to use at your normal times.

You should keep your reliever inhaler with you, and use it whenever you need to. However, you should let the nurses know that you have a reliever inhaler, and should inform them whenever you use it. This is because there is a possibility that it might interact with other treatments prescribed for you, and also so that they can keep an eye on how well your asthma is controlled.

Will the hospital be able to provide me with my special diet? I cannot eat eggs and milk.

When you first arrive at the hospital, you will be asked whether you have any special dietary requirements. The hospital kitchen will then be able to provide you with a suitable diet. They are well used to preparing food for people with special dietary needs, and should be able to provide you with everything you need. However, if there is a particular food or drink that you would really miss, take some with you or arrange for your visitors to come well supplied.

The last time I went into hospital my eczema became much worse. Why was this?

There are two reasons why your eczema may have become worse while you were in hospital. The first is that any hospital admission is a stressful experience, and stress almost always makes eczema worse. The second is that the sheets used on hospital beds are fairly heavy-duty and so can be quite rough, and they are also washed in strong chemical detergents and treated with starch. These chemical treatments are probably what irritated your skin. If you need to go into hospital again, ask if you may provide your own sheets.

I am very allergic to latex rubber, and have to go into hospital for an operation. Will the surgeon's gloves affect me?

There are a number of items used in hospitals which contain latex rubber, including the gloves worn by doctors and nurses during an operation. If you have a severe allergy to latex, it is important that you tell the surgeon and the rest of your health care team about it. They can then make sure that you are not exposed to items which contain latex.

I have suffered several anaphylactic reactions in the past, and I am very worried about having to go into hospital soon for an operation. What would happen if I had another reaction whilst under the anaesthetic? Would anyone notice?

I can understand your worry. When you are in hospital you could come into contact with a large number of products which could cause a serious allergic reaction, including anaesthetic drugs, antibiotics, products containing latex and foodstuffs containing peanut. You don't say what causes your anaphylactic reactions, but you probably know what it is. Explain that you have had these reactions and describe what caused them to the nurse who takes your details when you arrive on the ward, the doctors on the team looking after you and your anaesthetist (they will all be wearing name badges and should introduce themselves to you). They can then all make sure that you are not exposed to anything likely to set off a reaction during your stay.

It sounds as if you are worried that there might be other triggers which could set off your anaphylaxis, and that this could happen whilst you were anaesthetised. This is very unlikely, but if you were to suffer an allergic reaction during surgery, your anaesthetist (who never leaves you once you are asleep) would know about it very quickly. You are very closely monitored during an operation: any change in your heart rate and blood pressure would be noticed immediately, and treatment swiftly given.

Sex and pregnancy

My wife has a severe peanut allergy, but I adore peanuts. Could I be putting her at any risk if I continue to eat them?

Yes, you could, and there are two ways in which this could happen.

Firstly, if there are peanuts or foods containing peanuts in the house, there is always the possibility that she might accidentally eat something with peanuts in it, for example if biscuits containing peanuts inadvertently got mixed up with others in the same tin.

Secondly, if her peanut allergy is very severe, it is possible that she could develop an allergic reaction if enough peanut was passed to her from someone who has recently been eating peanuts, for example by you touching or kissing her after you have been eating them. People have been reported as having full blown anaphylactic reactions after a kiss on the lips from someone who has recently been eating peanuts.

For both these reasons it would make sense for peanuts to be banned from the house, and for you to think very carefully if you wish to continue to eat them. Your question provides a very good example of the way in which allergies can affect the whole family and not just the immediate sufferer.

Just recently my husband has quite literally been bringing me out in a rash! He has changed the brand of shaving cream and soap that he uses, and my eczema, which had been quite well controlled, now seems much worse. Is it possible that I am reacting to his toiletries?

In someone with extremely sensitive skin it is possible for this to happen, although it is not a common problem. I suggest you persuade your husband to go back to using the products which he used before and see whether, over a period of weeks, your eczema improves. If it does, then it is highly likely that your husband's new brand of toiletries were the cause of your problem.

I am allergic to latex, and both condoms and the contraceptive diaphragm give me a severe reaction. Any suggestions?

Most manufacturers now make special hypoallergenic condoms, which are available from most chemists. One of these is called 'Allergy', and is made by Durex. Not only are these made from non-allergenic materials, but they also have a water-based lubricant which does not contain a spermicide (something which can also cause an allergic reaction). I suggest you try these.

I get wheezy when I make love to my partner. Why is this, and what can I do about it?

There are a number of reasons why making love might make you wheezy. If exercise triggers your asthma, it might be that the physical exertion involved is making you wheezy. Emotion can be a powerful trigger for wheezing as well, so that might be part of your problem. Finally, it might be that your partner is using a perfume, aftershave, or other scented cosmetic which is making you wheeze. I suggest that you ask your partner to stop using any strongly perfumed preparations, and that you take two puffs of your reliever inhaler approximately 15 minutes before you make love. This may seem a little premeditated, but it should do the trick.

Will being pregnant make my asthma and other allergies worse?

The effect of pregnancy on asthma and other allergies is rather unpredictable. About half of the women with asthma who become pregnant find that the pregnancy has no effect on their asthma, and no change is needed in their medication. The other half experience a slight worsening of their asthma, requiring an increase in their anti-inflammatory treatment. Because the use of inhaled therapy allows such small doses to be taken, all asthma inhalers are perfectly safe to take during pregnancy. If you are using other medications for your other allergic problems then you should check with your doctor that it is safe to continue these during your pregnancy. All women with asthma should expect to have a normal pregnancy and a healthy baby.

There is no way of predicting exactly what will happen to your asthma while you are pregnant. If you feel that your symptoms are becoming worse, it is important that you consult your GP so that your treatment can be adjusted until your symptoms are back under control. This is because there is a small but real risk to your unborn baby if you were to have a severe asthma attack.

Can I use my usual asthma treatment whilst I'm pregnant?

Yes, you can. As a general rule, we advise that no drugs should be taken by mouth in the first four months of pregnancy, unless absolutely necessary. However, the use of inhaled therapy in asthma allows you to get the maximum benefit with the use of a very small dose. It is important that your asthma is well controlled during pregnancy, to avoid complications such as poor growth of your baby. You may find it helpful to monitor your peak flow recordings until your baby is born, so that you are aware of

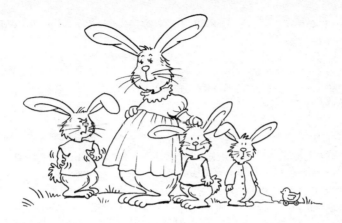

any deterioration in your asthma control (peak flow recordings and their use are discussed in the sections on *Diagnosis and assessment* in Chapter 2 and on *Peak expiratory flow testing* in Appendix 1).

I am worried that I may have an asthma attack during labour. Is this likely?

No, this is very unlikely. During labour, you produce high levels of two substances (cortisol and adrenaline), both of which are powerful anti-asthma agents. However, it will do no harm to you or your baby to use your reliever inhaler if you feel you need it.

Can I use my normal treatments for asthma and hayfever whilst I'm breast-feeding?

As a general rule, you can continue to take any treatment which is given directly into your lungs or nose by inhaler or spray without causing any problems for your baby. This is because such medications are taken in such small doses that very little, if any, will pass through to your breast milk. However, if you are taking antihistamines or any other types of medication by mouth, these may pass into your breast milk and could have an effect on your baby. It is therefore better to control your hayfever with sprays instead if you possibly can. Remind your doctor that you are breast-feeding so that any prescriptions can be adjusted if necessary.

Finance

Are people with allergies entitled to free prescriptions?

No. Needing medication regularly because you have an allergy does not qualify you for exemption from prescription charges. However, you may be exempt for other reasons – perhaps because of your age, or because you are pregnant, or because you have a very low income. A leaflet called *Are you entitled to help with health costs?* which will give you the details about this is available from your pharmacist.

If you are not exempt but still need a lot of prescriptions, then it may be worth considering pre-paying your prescription charges by buying a 'season ticket'. Before you go ahead and buy one, you will need to do a careful calculation based on the current price of ordinary prescriptions, the current price of the pre-payment certificate and your average number of prescriptions in a year to see whether it will be worth it for you. If you decide to go ahead, you will need to complete a form which is available from most doctors' surgeries, pharmacies and Post Offices.

I am finding the cost of the prescriptions for my severe eczema difficult to afford. I seem to require a large number of different medications, I am not entitled to free prescriptions, and I can't get enough money together at one time to buy a pre-payment certificate. What can I do?

Firstly, I suggest that you tell your doctor that you are having difficulty with the number of different treatments you require, as it may be possible to rationalise your treatment so as to decrease the number of different medications you need. This will not only make it cheaper for you, but could also make it easier for you to use them.

Secondly, there are many preparations (not just for eczema but for other allergies as well) which are cheaper to buy directly from your chemist than to obtain on prescription, as the cost is lower than the prescription charge. A considerable number of antihistamine tablets and syrups, nasal allergy sprays and anti-allergy eye drops, most emollients (moisturising and softening creams), and almost all emollient bath additives are cheaper to buy this way. Please don't feel embarrassed to discuss this with your GP, as doctors are well aware of this issue. All GPs receive a monthly publication, the *Drug and Therapeutics Bulletin*, which issues an annual supplement listing all the medicines which are cheaper to buy over the counter. You could also check with your pharmacist each time you fill a prescription that you are receiving your medications in the most economical way.

If you need a special diet because you have an allergy, can you get any help with the cost?

For infants who are allergic to cow's milk, a soya-based milk can be prescribed by a GP, and as the prescription is for a child, it will be free of charge. GPs can also prescribe all gluten-free foods for people with coeliac disease, although the regulations state that the doctor must be sure of the diagnosis and that the person concerned must be adequately monitored.

No other financial help is available for people with other allergic problems but, whatever the allergy, your modified diet need not be expensive. There are a number of special cookbooks for people with allergies, and more information about them can be obtained from the British Allergy Foundation (address in Appendix 2).

Miscellaneous

Should my daughter carry some sort of identification saying that she is allergic to peanuts?

This is a good idea, not just for children but also for adults who are at risk of, for example, anaphylaxis or severe asthma attacks. However careful you are about avoiding your allergy triggers, accidents can and do happen, and it may be vital that a medical emergency team knows about your condition. You can choose between an identity card or a piece of identification jewellery.

Identity cards usually have space to write in your personal details, your doctor's name and address, and some information about your allergy. They may be available from one of the self-help organisations (discussed later in this section) or your doctor may be able to provide you with one, as some of the pharmaceutical companies issue them free of charge. Obviously your daughter would always have to remember to carry it with her and not lose it. The other drawback is that people in this country are quite reserved and often will not look through someone's clothes or belongings for such a card.

Identification bracelets and necklaces are available from three companies – Golden Key, Medic-Alert and SOS Talisman (the addresses are in Appendix 2). Many people prefer them to identity cards as they are far more easily seen, more difficult to lose or forget, and by now most of the population knows that they exist and why. Styles vary: on some you need to have the details engraved, while others can be unscrewed to reveal a slip of paper containing the relevant information. The back-up provided by the companies also varies, and this may also affect your choice. For example, Medic-Alert (a non-profit-making charity established in 1965) keeps a computerised database of details of its members' medical conditions to which the emergency services have access.

Identification jewellery can be quite expensive, but if this is a problem you may be able to find a local voluntary organisation to help you. Several charities, including the Lions Club of Great Britain, support the Medic-Alert Foundation and in some cases will consider helping with the cost of joining the scheme. The Medic-Alert Foundation or your local library should be able to tell you how to make contact with the Lions if there is a club near you.

When should my son start being responsible for his own treatment? And how can I encourage him to do this?

The answer rather depends on how complicated your son's treatment is, but as a general rule I feel that most children from the age of five or six should be encouraged to become involved in their treatment in a very simple way, for example marking off doses taken on a wall chart, or putting together an asthma spacer device. By the age of seven, most children will be able to administer their own medication, but will still need help with remembering to take it.

The age at which a child becomes completely responsible for his or her own treatment will also depend on the child – some children can be fully independent by the age of 10, while others are still struggling at the age of 17! Many children will be encouraged to take on responsibility for their treatment themselves once they realise that doing so will give them much greater freedom, including the ability to stay overnight with friends, go on school trips, and so on.

The younger you can start your son's involvement with his treatment the better, and even very young children can take some sort of part.

I really resent the way that other people treat my allergies as something trivial. They don't seem to realise how difficult everyday things can be when you have these problems, and behave as if they just think I'm fussing about nothing. What can I do? I get miserable enough about my allergies without having to put up with this as well.

It must be very upsetting for you to feel that you do not have a great deal of support from your friends and family. I expect that the reason they behave like this is because they don't know very much about your allergic problems. Part of the difficulty probably lies in the fact that there is such a wide variety of allergic problems, and perhaps your friends mistakenly believe that all such problems are mild. You must also feel angry that your allergies stop you from leading a completely normal life.

The answer is probably to teach the people around you – your work colleagues as well as your family and friends – about your own allergic problems and how they affect you. You may find some of the educational leaflets from the British Allergy Foundation useful (the address is in Appendix 2), or some of the sections of this book may provide you with some of the information they need to know. Getting the facts across will not necessarily be easy, but the more people there are who are well informed about allergies, the easier the lives of those affected will be.

Are there any self-help or support groups for people with allergies?

Yes, there are, and you will find details of a number of them in Appendix 2. The services provided by these organisations vary depending on their size and the amount of funding they receive, but most offer local meetings of support groups, information packs, magazines and telephone helplines, and many also support research. If you cannot find a specific support group for your particular allergic problem, I suggest you contact the British Allergy Foundation, which offers help for all people with allergies.

Allergen avoidance and complementary therapies

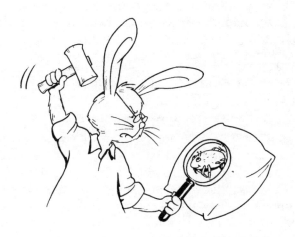

Introduction

Perhaps the best treatment of all for an allergy is completely to avoid whatever it is that sets off the symptoms. In this chapter I describe some practical ways in which you can reduce your contact with the allergens which are responsible for several different types of allergy, ie those that make most people's problems worse. Allergens and triggers which are specific to individual allergies are discussed in the chapters relating to those particular allergies.

Not all allergens can be avoided. If you are allergic to one which is unavoidable, medications are available which can usually help to prevent or relieve symptoms (these treatments have also been discussed in earlier chapters). Conventional medical therapy cannot, as yet, provide a cure for allergies, but instead aims to keep symptoms under control by reducing the inflammation which is at the root of all allergic problems, and by making the body less susceptible to the trigger factors which can set off an attack. However, many people dislike taking medications regularly, and find therapies which do not involve drug treatments far more attractive. The final section of this chapter looks at these complementary therapies, and discusses which of them might be of particular benefit to you.

Allergen avoidance in general

Which are the most troublesome allergens?

The allergens responsible for causing the most symptoms are probably the aero-allergens, that is those which are carried in the air. The most important aero-allergens are the house dust mite, pollens from grass and trees, and the pet allergens, and there are sections on all of these in this chapter. Foodstuffs can also cause problems: although true food allergy (discussed in Chapter 5) is not very common, some foods can act as trigger factors for other allergies, which is why there is a section on them in this chapter.

My daughter has such problems with her allergies that my husband and I would be prepared to move if it would help. Are allergies more common in certain parts of the country, and where would be best for my daughter?

Allergies occur wherever there are allergens, and in this country that means almost everywhere. However, the amount of allergen in an area can be dependent – at least to some extent – on local environmental, meteorological and geographical features. For example, hayfever can show a definite geographical variation because of differences in the airborne pattern of pollen distribution, and this is why details of the pollen count given in the local media are often more accurate and useful than any national figures.

Allergens are less common at high altitude. Not only are there fewer lush pollen-producing plants and trees, but the house dust mite is less common too, as it thrives in warm humid conditions and dislikes the cool dry air found in mountainous areas. Unfortunately, if you want to take advantage of this you will need to move abroad, as nowhere in the United Kingdom reaches the altitude needed to reduce the levels of the house dust mite.

Factors other than allergens also need to be considered. For example, polluted air is not itself an allergen, but it can aggravate an existing allergy. Moving from a rural to a built-up area might reduce someone's exposure to a particular plant allergen, but the effect of higher pollution levels might then cancel out any benefit gained. Conversely, moving to an area with lower air pollution might remove an aggravating factor, but could lead to exposure to a new trigger not previously encountered while living in a large town or city.

As you can see, there is no easy answer to your question, and moving house will not necessarily be helpful. This does not mean that there are not ways to make life easier for your daughter. Many allergies (especially those associated with asthma) are more affected by the indoor environment than by outdoor factors. I think you would be better off finding out to which allergens your daughter is allergic (your doctor can arrange for her to have tests of the types described in Appendix 1), and then doing whatever you can to make your home, and in particular your daughter's bedroom, as free from these allergens as possible.

Allergies run in my family. Is there anything that I can do to prevent my children developing allergies?

This is a very interesting and important question. There probably are a number of things that parents can do to prevent their children developing allergies – asthma in particular – but at the moment we do not have full scientific proof that they work. We will have to wait for the results of research studies in this area before we can recommend these measures. However, I can give you an idea of the areas which are being investigated.

- **Diet**
  Early exposure of a baby to foodstuffs which are known to be associated with allergy may be a contributing factor to the development of allergic problems. The exclusion of cow's milk and hen's eggs from a child's diet until the age of one year may be helpful. It might prove to be even more important to avoid exposing an unborn baby to these foodstuffs before birth, and that would mean the mother avoiding them in her own diet during pregnancy. And remember, animal proteins can find their way into human breast milk, and so these foods would have to be avoided by a breast-feeding mother if she wished to protect her baby from them.

- **Aero-allergens**
  Allergens light enough to be carried in the air and inhaled are called aero-allergens. Early exposure to aero-allergens such as animal dander (for example cat and dog hair), grass pollens and the house dust mite may increase the risk of a baby developing allergies. In the case of pollens, this risk has been shown to be higher in infants born just before and during the main pollen season (April to July in the United Kingdom) and who are therefore exposed to higher levels of pollen whilst very young than those born at other times of the year. We also know that babies born into a household with a cat are at least twice as likely to develop asthma than a baby from a cat-free home.

- **Tobacco smoke**
  Children of women who smoke experience passive exposure to tobacco smoke both before birth (via the placenta) and in early childhood. There is absolutely no question that this increases their chances of developing asthma. It also increases the risk of other respiratory diseases. Pregnant women, babies and children should NEVER be exposed to tobacco smoke.

House dust mite

I'm far from being the world's best at housework. Is the house dust mite really so important that I should start making an effort to keep the dust levels down?

For most people with allergies, the answer is yes, although dusting and vacuuming are only part of the solution. Allergy to house dust mite is the commonest allergy in this country, affecting 80% of all adults and children with asthma. It also affects people with perennial allergic rhinitis and eczema. However, before you spend time, money and energy trying to eradicate house dust mites from your home, you should discover whether or not you are allergic to them. If you are not, there is no point in trying to avoid them. Your doctor can arrange for you to be skin prick tested if there is any doubt about it (skin prick testing is explained in Appendix 1).

House dust is made up of an enormous number of different things, including fibres from fabrics, lint, food particles, skin scales from humans and from animals, hair, and millions of microscopically small creatures, too small to be seen with the naked eye. The house dust mite (shown in Figure 12) is the most common of these creatures. Its Latin name is *Dermatophagoides pteronyssinus*, and it is found in almost all of our homes, where it feeds off the skin scales found in house dust.

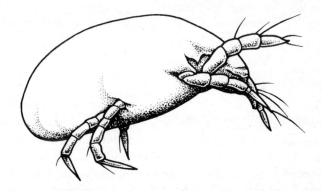

Figure 12: House dust mite, shown 500 times actual size.

The number of house dust mites in your home will not vary a great deal throughout the year, although it will tend to be a little higher in autumn and winter. The mites thrive in warm humid conditions, liking best a temperature of around 25°C and a relative humidity of about 80% (conditions found in most centrally-heated houses), although they are capable of living in cooler and drier places. The house dust mite is rare in very cold countries and at high altitude, and house dust mite allergy is not a significant factor in the development of asthma, eczema and allergic rhinitis in such places. Because of this, children who are allergic to the house dust mite show an improvement in their asthma when they spend prolonged periods of time at high altitudes.

Assuming that we can't all move to the mountains, how can we reduce the levels of house dust mite in our homes? Firstly we must look at where the house dust mite lives. The warm humid conditions that the mites like are found in the insides of mattresses, in pillows, in carpets and curtains, and in cuddly toys. Secondly we must look at what part of the mite causes the problem. It is not actually the mite itself to which we are allergic, but its droppings. This means that even if we were able to kill all of the mites, allergy problems would continue unless we were also able to remove all of the mite faecal pellets. Thirdly we must look at how the mite allergen causes problems. It is only when our lungs, our nasal passages, or our skin comes into contact with the mite allergen that symptoms are produced. If we could put a barrier between us and the allergen, we would be protected from getting symptoms.

The practical steps that you can take to reduce your exposure to the house dust mite allergen are discussed in the remaining answers in this section.

Do I need to buy a new vacuum cleaner?

Not necessarily, it will depend on the model you already own and how effective it is. To reduce house dust mite levels, you really need to use a high-efficiency vacuum cleaner fitted with a special filter which has a pore size of less than 0.3 micrometres. Many ordinary domestic vacuum cleaners are now fitted with this type of filter, and these can be just as effective as the more expensive 'medical' vacuum cleaners. You can find information about each vacuum cleaner model direct from the manufacturers or from the shops selling them. Alternatively, contact the British Allergy Foundation (address in Appendix 2) which organises independent tests on many products, including vacuum cleaners, and can provide lists of those which perform to set standards.

The bedroom and living room should be vacuumed daily, and preferably when the person with the allergy is not in the room (if you have the allergy yourself, then you should try to find someone to do the vacuuming for you). The machine should be emptied regularly (again you may need to ask someone to do this for you), and the filters replaced according the manufacturer's instructions. As well as vacuuming the carpets, it is worth vacuuming your mattress each time you change the sheets, as although this won't remove all the mites, it will help to keep the numbers down.

I've been advised that reducing the amount of house dust mite in my bedding will help my eczema. Is this true, and if so, what should I do?

Yes, your eczema may be significantly improved by reducing the levels of house dust mite in your bedroom, in particular in your mattress and bedding. While you are in bed, your skin is in close contact with very high levels of the house dust mite allergen, which can be particularly troublesome if your skin is inflamed or broken.

The following suggestions apply not just to people with eczema, but to anyone allergic to the house dust mite – after all, we spend more of our lives in the bedroom than in any other single place, and approximately one-third of our lives in bed, so it is an obvious starting place for reducing levels of this allergen. Which of these measures you will need to adopt will depend on the severity of your allergy – I suggest you start with the simplest and cheapest first, and only go on to such things as replacing furniture and carpets if it proves necessary.

In addition, I suggest that you do not allow any pets in the bedroom (especially not on the bed). Not only can the house dust

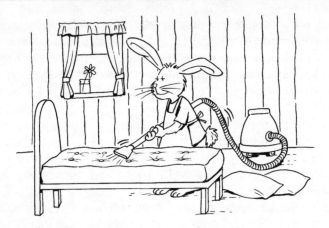

mite feed on animal dander, but also because pets themselves can be major sources of allergens. There is a section on **Pet allergens** later in this chapter.

- **Vacuuming**
  Vacuum regularly with a high efficiency vacuum cleaner fitted with an effective filter (as described in the answer to the previous question). As well as the carpet, vacuum the mattress, the curtains and any soft furnishings such as padded headboards and upholstered chairs.

- **Bedding**
  Wash all your bedding (including pillows, duvets and blankets) regularly at as high a temperature as possible (60°C or higher is best). Air it regularly as well, preferably in direct sunlight.

- **Pillows and duvets**
  If you currently have feather or down pillows and duvets, consider replacing them with new ones made from synthetic fibres rather than natural fillings, as feathers can themselves be the cause of allergies. Synthetics also have the advantage that they can be washed regularly.

- **Barrier covers**
  Most of the house dust mite in bedrooms comes from mattresses and pillows. The simplest way to tackle these items is by enclosing them in covers which do not allow the house

dust mite or its droppings to escape. They act as a barrier between you and the mites.

The cheapest solution is to use plastic mattress and pillow covers. These should be of the type which completely enclose the mattress and pillows, and the zip fastenings should be sealed up with adhesive tape. Plastic sheets are nowhere near as effective, because they do not cover the whole mattress, so allowing dust to escape from the bottom. The disadvantages of these plastic covers is that they are uncomfortable, as they become quite hot and damp, and they are also noisy when you turn over in bed.

A more expensive but much more comfortable alternative is to use a system of anti-allergy covers made from one of the microporous materials which are 'breathable'. These allow air to circulate, but are so tightly woven that the house dust mite and its droppings cannot escape. The British Allergy Foundation (address in Appendix 2) can provide you with information on manufacturers, and will also tell you which of these products have the BAF's seal of approval, that is those which in independent testing conform to certain set standards.

I would recommend that you ask the advice of your doctor before you buy these covers, and that you only purchase them if tests have proved you to be allergic to the house dust mite. They will be a waste of quite a lot of money if you are not. If you decide to go for this option, you must use the whole system, which will include a duvet cover as well as mattress and pillow covers.

- **Cuddly toys**
  Ideally, cuddly toys should not be kept in the bedroom. If toys have to be stored in the bedroom, they should be put in a cupboard or a plastic box with a lid. If a child has a favourite cuddly toy without which he or she cannot sleep, then it should be washed once a week at a temperature of at least 60°C. Alternatively, once a week the toy should be put in a plastic bag and then placed in a freezer for at least six hours (intense cold kills the house dust mite). It must be then vacuumed to remove the dead mites and their droppings.

- **Beds**
  If possible, avoid sleeping in a bed with a divan base (which itself can be an ideal home for the house dust mite), and use a bed with a slatted base instead. Avoid bunk-beds and beds with canopies, as these can shower dust and mite allergen down onto the person sleeping underneath.

  Beds and items of upholstered furniture can now be heat treated: the item to be treated is enclosed in a plastic cover, and the air inside the cover is heated to 100°C. This both kills the house dust mite and changes the protein in the droppings to make it non-allergenic. This service is provided by a company called Sleepsafe Systems, whose address is given in Appendix 2.

- **Upholstery and soft furnishings**
  Padded headboards, upholstered chairs and other soft furnishings provide perfect conditions for the house dust mite, so you may want to consider removing them from the bedroom. If you decide to keep them, they will need regular vacuuming. Curtains should be plain cotton, preferably unlined, and washed regularly. Roller blinds are a good alternative.

- **Carpets**
  If you want to have bedroom carpets, then those made from synthetic fibres are preferable to those made from wool. Synthetics allow less house dust mite allergen to escape into the air because of a static charge which keeps the mite particles down in the carpet. However, it would be better to have a hardwood or lino flooring, as these do not harbour the house dust mite and are easier to clean.

- **Humidity and ventilation**
  Try to reduce the humidity inside the bedroom by improving ventilation as much as possible. The easiest and cheapest way to do this is to open the windows! If you are allergic to pollen, then in your pollen season you should only open the windows in the late evening and during the night, when pollen levels are lowest. Although in theory ionisers and dehumidifiers should

decrease the numbers of house dust mites in the home, as yet there is relatively little scientific proof to show this. I would suggest that you try other measures first before buying these relatively expensive pieces of equipment.

- **House dust mite sprays**
  Sprays which kill the house dust mite are called acaracide sprays, and there are a number of them on the market. They are only able to penetrate a few millimetres into furnishings, which means that they are therefore not very effective on bulky items, although they might be of use on carpets. I would not recommend that you use these sprays on your bed or bedding for several reasons: they do not penetrate well into the centre of the mattress and so do not kill all the house dust mites; they do not actually remove house dust mite allergen already in the mattress; and the chemicals they contain can irritate some people's eyes and skin.

What about other rooms in the house apart from the bedrooms?

The next most important room to tackle after the bedroom is probably the living room, but don't forget about any other rooms where you may spend a great deal of your time, such as a home office or a children's playroom. With a little adaptation where necessary, the suggestions I have given for controlling house dust mites in the bedroom apply equally well to the other rooms in the house.

I am considering buying a new home with a heating system which consists of a warm air unit blowing hot air through ducts from a central heating source to all the rooms. Is this advisable in light of the fact that I am allergic to house dust mite?

This is the worst style of heating you could have! However much you try to keep the house dust mite in your home under control, it is impossible to eradicate it completely. The type of heating you describe will constantly blow the dust containing the house dust mite allergen up into the air where you will breathe it in. It is the levels of mite and mite allergen in the air which matter most, and any device which actively blows air around will lead to increased levels of air-borne dust mite. For this reason, fan heaters and convector heaters are not advisable either. The least troublesome form of heating for people with allergies is gas central heating using radiators and with the gas boiler well away from the living area.

Pollens

Why is pollen such a problem?

Pollens are the male reproductive cells of plants and trees. Pollen grains are very small and very light, so that they can be carried by insects or by the wind to reach other trees or plants of the same species and fertilise them. The pollen carried by insects is not usually a problem for people with allergies, as it is heavier and less likely to become airborne, but wind-borne pollen is. Wind pollination is not a very efficient way of fertilisation, and so the plants have to produce many millions of pollen grains. These are so light and dry that large quantities of them can be carried in the air for many miles. This makes pollen very difficult to avoid, as you will know if you have hayfever or pollen-induced asthma.

I've heard of pollen calendars but I have no idea what they are. How will one help me?

Different plants and trees produce their flowers and their pollens at different times of year, and a pollen calendar shows you approximately when to expect these pollens to be released into the air. An example is shown in Figure 13.

If you have a pollen allergy, the time of year when your symptoms occur will depend on the release of the pollen or pollens which are your particular triggers. If you know which pollens trigger your allergy, then you can use a pollen calendar to warn you when to expect trouble. If you don't, but can remember when your symptoms start each year, then the calendar might help you identify the pollen or pollens responsible. In either case,

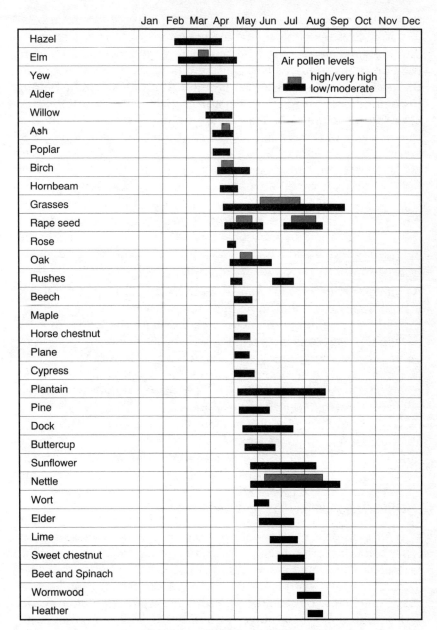

Figure 13: Pollen calendar.

your hayfever treatment will be most effective if begun at least two to four weeks before you expect your symptoms to start.

A pollen calendar can be a useful guide, but you need to remember that unusual weather conditions can advance or delay the pollen season a little. In addition, the pollen count on any particular day will vary according to the weather and atmospheric conditions occurring that day. The pollen count is the measure of the number of pollen grains carried in one cubic metre of air. A count of below 50 is regarded as low, and one over 200 as very high. Unfortunately, if you are allergic to a particular pollen, even a low count can produce severe symptoms.

Everyone else seems to look forward to summer, but I dread it because I know that my allergies are going to be at their very worst. What can I do to make my life more bearable during the pollen season?

As I have said before, the most effective way of treating an allergy is completely to avoid the responsible allergen. In pollen allergy, the only way of doing this would be to spend the whole of your personal pollen season in a place where the responsible plant or plants do not grow, which might be a long way away from home. Not many of us can afford to do this (nor would we really want to), and there would always be the chance that you would develop a new allergy to a different pollen. This means that the mainstay of pollen allergy treatment is to take medications, such as antihistamine nasal sprays and tablets, and other anti-inflammatory treatments as prescribed by your doctor in order to suppress your symptoms. There are, however, some commonsense measures you can take to reduce your exposure to pollen and so make your summers more enjoyable.

- Spend as little time as possible out of doors on days and at times of day when the pollen count is high, for example in the late afternoon and early evening on fine sunny days.
- Time outdoor exercise and sporting activities such as jogging and tennis for those periods of the day when the pollen count is likely to be at its lowest, such as the early morning, late evening or after a rain shower.

- Wearing glasses may reduce symptoms that affect your eyes, so use spectacles instead of contact lenses, or consider wearing sunglasses when you are outside.
- If you have been out of doors when the pollen count was high, change your clothes when you come indoors again.
- Keep the doors and windows of your house closed during the day to keep the pollen out.
- If possible, arrange your holiday for the height of your pollen season and go away. Consider taking your holidays in coastal areas where sea breezes keep the air relatively pollen-free, or going abroad to a country where your particular pollen trigger is unlikely to occur.
- Dry your washing indoors (preferably in a tumble-drier) rather than outdoors, as clothes and bedding can trap pollen grains.
- Avoid mowing the lawn – get someone else to cut the grass! Don't handle newly cut grass.
- Consider buying an air-intake filter for your car or, if you are buying a new car, choose one with a pollen filter already fitted to the ventilation system. These filters are becoming more readily available, and can now been found in smaller cars as well as expensive luxury models.
- Avoid all the other things such as smoke, dust and traffic fumes which will make your symptoms worse.

I'm a keen gardener, so how can I reduce my exposure to pollen?

You are far from being alone in asking this question. In response to this type of request, a low allergen garden was created for the National Asthma Campaign and exhibited at the Chelsea Flower Show. Contact the Campaign at the address in Appendix 2 for further details. You might also find the following suggestions helpful.

- Consult the pollen forecast before going out of doors. A pollen count of 50 or above will be likely to bring on your symptoms.
- Do your gardening on cold, wet or dull days. Grass flowers do not open or release their pollen on dull or wet days. In addition, rain washes the pollen out of the atmosphere.

- Do your gardening first thing in the morning when the pollen count is at its lowest. Cool damp mornings – especially when there is dew – will cause the fewest symptoms.
- Don't do your gardening on days when the air quality is poor. Pollution adds greatly to the irritant effects of pollen.
- Try wearing sunglasses while you are out in the garden. These reduce the circulation of air which carries the pollen grains around your eyes. Tight-fitting glasses with large lenses are the best.
- Consider having decorative paving or gravel instead of a lawn. If you decide to have a lawn, then get someone else to cut it and dispose of the clippings, and make sure it is cut regularly so that the grasses do not get the chance to flower.
- Choose plants which are insect-pollinated rather than wind-pollinated.
- Don't grow allergen-producing plants such as birch trees, ornamental grasses and members of the daisy family.
- Don't forget that weeds can be just as much a problem as cultivated plants. Control them by regular weeding or, preferably, by mulching or growing ground-cover plants.

A very useful booklet called *Hayfever in the Garden* is available from Hoechst Marion Roussel: details of how to obtain a copy are given in Appendix 3.

Pet allergens

Which pets cause the most problems for people with allergies?

The most common animal allergy in the United Kingdom is to cats, but dogs, horses, rabbits and birds also cause problems. We are a nation of animal lovers, and between 60% and 80% of households have a pet of some kind. When you consider that as many as a third of all atopic people are allergic to animals, you can see that they are a major trigger factor. For example, a recent study has shown that exposure to pet allergen may be at least partly responsible for causing over 40% of all childhood asthma in the UK. Infants and small children are particularly at risk of becoming sensitized to pet allergens, and should be protected from contact with furry animals.

If you are allergic to animals, wouldn't just avoiding stroking or playing with them be enough to prevent them causing you problems?

Unfortunately not. Animals produce allergens in a number of different ways: their hair and skin is allergenic, so shed fur and skin scales (dander) are a major source, but the allergens are also present in saliva, urine and faeces (droppings). It is not necessary to handle an animal to come into contact with an allergen – animal allergens can travel in the air, and can also be passed from person to person by way of clothing, and even by sitting on the same chair.

Animal allergens can quickly become widely spread around the home. If you or another member of your family are allergic to animals and you already have or want to buy a pet, it is not sufficient to restrict the pet to one room of the house or just to the downstairs. Wherever the pet lives the allergen will be spread around the house by the rest of the family, and the allergic person will be just as exposed as if the pet was living in the whole house.

In fact, it is not even necessary to own a pet to become sensitized. Animal allergens are so potent that you can meet enough of them during your everyday contact with other people to become allergic. For example, even sitting on a bus seat which has been used by an animal owner can bring on some people's symptoms.

Animal allergens can stay around for a long time. If the previous owner of your house or car had a pet, it will take a long period of regular cleaning before every trace of allergen disappears. Six months of hard work with an efficient vacuum cleaner is needed before a house can be said to be free of cat allergens.

How do I know that it really is our dog which is causing the

problems? I don't want to have to find him another home unless I really have to.

Many people think that if you are allergic to a pet you will suffer acute attacks of your asthma or eczema or rhinitis, and that because of this the allergy will be obvious. In fact, this is rarely the case. Instead, the constant exposure to the allergen keeps your allergy ticking over, making your general condition worse but not producing obvious attacks. If you want to know for sure whether you are allergic to a particular animal (your dog in your case), then skin prick testing or RAST might make this clearer. Your doctor can arrange these tests, which are described in Appendix 1.

You could also try sending your dog away for a 'holiday' (perhaps a friend or relative will take him) to see whether this affects your symptoms. The dog will have to be sent away for at least six months, to give you time to clear most of the allergen from the house and to allow your symptoms time to improve.

Our son is allergic to our cat, but is so distressed at the thought that she might have to go to another home that we have decided to keep her. What can we do to try to keep the allergen level down?

This is a common problem as, like many other people, you consider your pet to be a member of your family with whom you would not be prepared to part. The following suggestions may help, but they will not solve the problem completely.

- Can the cat live outside if you provide her with suitable shelter? She should then not be allowed into the house at all. You will need to keep special clothes to wear when grooming her, and you should not bring these into the house either.
- It is said that shampooing a cat every week reduces the amount of allergen it sheds – although this might turn out to be one piece of advice which is easier said than done.
- Use a high-efficiency vacuum cleaner (as described in the earlier section on *House dust mite*), and use it regularly to remove as much of the allergen in the house as possible.
- Try to keep your son's contact with the cat to the minimum

which will not cause him additional distress – if necessary, he should change his clothes when he comes into the house after playing with her outside.

I think that it is good for children to have pets, but I see the problem about allergies. What pets could we have?

Consider a pet which does not shed allergen, such as fish, or one which is kept in a cage and therefore is not free to spread allergen around the house, such as a hamster or a gerbil. These have the added advantages of being cheap to keep and not needing long walks! Alternatively, why not arrange for your child to adopt an animal at your local zoo or wildlife park? This makes an excellent present, need not be expensive, and a wide range of species are available.

Food allergens

Foods of different types seem to be blamed for most things these days – are they really such a problem in allergies as some people make out?

Certainly some people have a true allergy to certain foods (as discussed in Chapter 5), and for them there is no doubt that eating particular foodstuffs presents real problems. When it comes to other types of allergy, then the role played by foodstuffs is debatable.

It has been suggested that certain foods and food additives might be responsible for both causing and maintaining a number of allergies (including asthma, eczema and bowel problems), as well as perhaps being implicated in other less clearly defined problems. Although as many as 50% of young children and 30% of adults with asthma and eczema may react to food allergens on skin prick testing, most doctors do not believe that these foods represent the main cause of their asthma or eczema. Individuals who develop these allergies do so because they have an inherited tendency to allergies called atopy (this is discussed in more detail in the section on *Allergy explained* in Chapter 1). Once they have developed an allergy, they are then capable of reacting to a number of things, including foods. Avoiding a particular food will not solve the whole problem, and only in a few people will an elimination or exclusion diet significantly decrease the symptoms.

Unfortunately, many people wrongly blame food allergy for a wide range of symptoms, including behavioural problems and sleep disorders in children. As a result they needlessly limit their choice of foods, their lifestyle and their enjoyment of life by continuing on a special diet. It is important to realise that there are a number of other factors which might be responsible for your allergy symptoms, and you should only exclude foods if it is appropriate. In this case, 'appropriate' means after talking the matter through with your doctor and confirming using the correct tests that a particular food really does affect you in the way you suspect.

Who can benefit from food avoidance?

People with true food allergies will benefit by excluding the foods which trigger their symptoms from their diet, and people with food intolerance or food sensitivity (neither of which are allergies) may also need or want to avoid certain foods. These topics are all discussed in Chapter 5.

In other people, specific food avoidance is unlikely to lead to an improvement in their allergies. The exceptions are young children with eczema, and people with asthma who also have other allergic problems such as urticaria (urticaria is discussed in the section on *Skin allergies explained* in Chapter 3).

Which foods cause the most problems?

The foods to which people are most frequently allergic include the following:

- cow's milk;
- eggs;
- peanuts (which are not actually nuts at all);
- true nuts (also called tree nuts);
- shellfish;

- white fish;
- wheat;
- corn;
- bananas; and
- citrus fruit.

If I do need to exclude a food from my diet, how do I go about doing it?

Only one food at a time should be excluded from your diet and then only when there is good reason to believe that that food might be the cause of the problem. If no improvement occurs, then the food should be replaced before another is excluded. Children should not be put on elimination or exclusion diets of any sort unless you have discussed it first with your doctor: children need the nutrients found in a comprehensive range of foodstuffs to be able to grow well and develop normally.

If you have been found to be allergic to a particular food, you will need to exclude it completely from your diet. This can be difficult, as packaged, pre-prepared and convenience foods sometimes contain some surprising ingredients. You will need to read all food labels very carefully, and develop the knack of spotting all the different names under which particular ingredients can be listed. Remember too that manufacturers sometimes change the ingredients they use without any warning, so you must read the packet labels each and every time you buy a food, whether or not you have used it before. I would also suggest that you consult a dietician for specialist advice.

To give you some idea of just what will be involved, here are some (but not all) of the foods you would need to avoid on three common types of exclusion diet.

- **Milk-free diets**
  You must not only avoid drinking milk (whether whole, semi-skimmed or skimmed) but also avoid it in all foodstuffs. This means avoiding foods which contain any of the following: milk;

whey; casein; caseinates; lactose; dried milk solids; and milk
powder.

Foods made from or containing milk include the following:
cream; butter; cheese; yoghurt; fromage frais; crème fraîche;
condensed milk; evaporated milk; most ice creams; most
margarines and low-fat spreads; milk chocolate; and desserts
such as rice puddings. You should also avoid any foodstuffs
that contain any of the foods on this list as ingredients.

Most breads, cakes and biscuits are prepared with milk, as
are ready-made or powdered soups and sauces. Breakfast
cereals and muesli often contain milk powder. When it comes
to drinks, you will need to avoid coffee creamers, malted milk
drinks such as Ovaltine, drinking chocolate and 'instant'
chocolate-based drinks.

- **Egg-free diets**
You must not only avoid eating eggs (however they are
prepared) but also all foodstuffs containing egg in any form.
This means avoiding foods which contain any of the following:
egg; egg white; dried egg; and albumen.

The following foods usually contain egg: custard; puddings;
ice creams; chocolate; noodles; fried rice; cakes; biscuits;
meringues; pancakes; batter puddings such as Yorkshire
pudding; sauces; and mayonnaise and salad cream.

Remember that eggs can often be used as glazing on baked
goods.

- **Wheat-free diets**
Avoiding wheat means avoiding any of the following: wheat;
flour; starch; bran; wheatgerm; durum wheat; and semolina.

The following foods usually contain wheat: bread; most
biscuits (whether sweet or savoury); most cereals; most pasta
and noodles; breadcrumbs and foods containing breadcrumbs
such as sausages and hot dogs; and any sauces, soups or gravy
thickened with flour.

Remember that breads and biscuits made from other grains
such as rye and corn usually contain some wheat as well.

Complementary therapies

What's your opinion on people with allergies using complementary therapies?

First of all, I would like to make a distinction between medicines or therapies which claim to be 'alternatives' to treatments offered by the medical profession, and those which claim to be 'complementary', which their practitioners intend to be used alongside conventional treatments. No one should stop taking their prescribed allergy treatments without first consulting their doctor, and I would suggest that you avoid any 'alternative' practitioners who tell you that their therapies will not work unless you give up your usual medication. Complementary treatments offer their greatest benefits when used hand-in-hand with conventional treatment, and reputable complementary practitioners recognise this (finding such reputable practitioners is discussed in the answer to the next question).

Some doctors are rather dismissive of complementary therapies, saying that they have not been proved to work, and therefore discourage their patients from using them. Other doctors take the attitude that these therapies may be a useful help to relaxation, but for little else. My own opinion is that there is still a great deal that is not yet known about the treatment of allergy, and that provided they do no harm and are used wisely, complementary therapies may be of some benefit to certain people with allergies. After all, stress, excitement and anxiety can all trigger allergies or make them seem worse, so relaxation is no bad thing!

I would emphasise that these therapies should be used at the same time as the treatments prescribed by your doctor, which should never be stopped suddenly as this could be dangerous. In addition, complementary treatments should never be relied upon at the time of an emergency. Acute attacks of asthma and other allergies should always be managed by fully qualified doctors using conventional treatments. Remember that many complementary therapists have no formal medical training, and might not be able to recognise certain important complications of your illness.

How can I make sure that I pick a decent therapist and not a quack?

This can be difficult. In this country complementary therapies are virtually unregulated – very different from the position in the rest of Europe, where registration of practitioners is compulsory in many countries, with only registered health professionals being allowed to practice.

However, there are a number of organisations representing complementary therapy practitioners in the United Kingdom: usually each therapy has its own 'governing body' and there are also umbrella organisations trying to improve standards across the whole range of complementary treatments. You will find the relevant addresses listed in the *HEA Guide to Complementary Medicine and Therapies* (details in Appendix 3) and you could write to them to ask for names of qualified practitioners in your area. I suggest you also ask around locally for recommendations. Your GP may know of reputable practitioners in your area, and some health centres now offer some complementary therapies themselves.

Before you start on a course of a complementary therapy, I suggest that you ask the following questions, and only agree to go ahead with it if you are satisfied with the answers you receive.

- What are the therapist's qualifications?
- How long was their training and how long have they been practising?
- Is the therapist registered with a recognised organisation?
- What is their attitude to conventional medicine?
- Will the therapist contact your GP?
- What does the treatment involve?
- Is it the most appropriate therapy for your condition?
- How many sessions will you need?
- What will they cost?
- Is the treatment available on the NHS?

You should be very wary of any therapist who claims to be able to cure you.

I have heard that acupuncture can be useful for people

with allergies. Is this true? I would be interested in trying it if I didn't dislike needles so much. Is it as painful as it sounds? Are there any similar treatments that don't use needles?

Acupuncture is a therapy based on traditional Chinese methods, in which fine needles are inserted at specific points of the body to stimulate energy flow and to restore equilibrium in the body. The Chinese believe that our life-force (which they call 'chi') functions by the flow of energy through clearly defined channels in the body (these are called meridians), and that a blockage in this energy flow results in illness. Diagnosis is not based on patterns of specific symptoms as it is in Western medicine, but on a wider assessment of the individual's mood, character and life situation.

Acupuncture may be used for a wide range of reasons including pain relief, anaesthesia for operations, to help someone give up smoking, and for the treatment of asthma. Although in asthma it has been shown to produce relaxation of the airways and a temporary increase in peak flow, it has not been shown to be of long-term benefit. Chinese clinics treat people with asthma

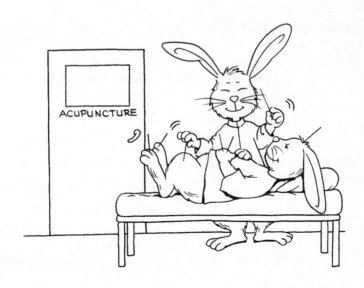

on a daily basis over very long periods of time: in this country that would be very expensive and would not seem to offer any advantage over conventional treatments. Acupuncture is sometimes used in other allergies such as hayfever.

At the beginning of the session, the acupuncturist will make notes on your medical problems, and will examine the pulses on each wrist. Very fine stainless steel needles will then be inserted into your skin at a number of points on your body, the exact number and position depending on the acupuncturist's assessment of the treatment you require. The needles will be left in place for from 5-30 minutes, and may or may not be connected to a device called an electro-stimulator. The needle insertion is virtually painless, and produces no bleeding.

As you dislike needles so much, you could consider shiatsu as an alternative. This therapy developed at the same time as acupuncture, and works using the same energy system of meridians. Instead of needles, gentle pressure is applied to the acupuncture points. However, it is more of a general therapy to induce relaxation and well-being rather than one intended to treat specific illnesses.

As aromatherapy uses oils made from plants, can it be used by people with allergies?

As you say, aromatherapy involves treatment with essential oils, which are aromatic (scented) oils extracted from the roots, flowers or leaves of plants by distillation. It can be used by people with allergies, and indeed has been used to treat people with allergies such as asthma and eczema. It is very unusual for people to be allergic to the pure essential oils used at the correct dilution.

A fully-qualified practitioner (you should avoid aroma-therapists who are only qualified to give beauty treatments) will ask you about your allergies and will only use oils which will not trigger your symptoms. The oils are chosen so as to balance your body systems. The aromatherapist will make you up your own prescription of oils and give you suggestions on how you can use them at home (in the bath, perhaps, or as an inhalation).

An aromatherapy treatment often involves massage, which in

itself can be very relaxing. It may help to relieve any tensions and stresses which might be making your allergies worse.

What about other types of massage – are they of any use?

If stress triggers your allergy or makes it worse, then anything which helps you relax may be useful, and most forms of massage are very relaxing.

One type of massage which is thought to help in asthma (although there is no scientific proof of this) is reflexology, a form of foot massage. The foot is divided into zones which represent the organs of the body. Energy lines or zones are considered to run up and down the feet, connecting the different organs. Massage of the various zones of the foot are claimed to help specific illnesses as well as restoring general well-being. It may simply be of help by being relaxing – providing you are not ticklish!

There has been a lot of publicity about people whose eczema has been cured by using Chinese herbs. Is this really effective, and will herbal medicine help anyone with an allergy?

Herbal medicines have been used for thousands of years, and the medicinal properties of a number of these substances have been confirmed by scientific research. Herbal medicines are made from the leaves, roots, flowers or bark of plants. Although they are regarded as a complementary treatment in this country, some 60% of the world's population uses no other form of medicine. Side effects are rare.

Medical herbalists take a broad or holistic approach to treatment, aiming to use herbal treatments to improve general well-being as well as to reduce specific symptoms. Herbal remedies are used in combinations which are chosen specifically for each individual and their problems. For an allergy herbalists would aim to give you remedies which would strengthen your immune system and so make you react less strongly to your particular triggers, but a reputable practitioner will not claim to be able to cure you of all your symptoms.

The form of Chinese herbal medicine you mention has appeared to be very effective in certain cases of eczema, and is currently being formally assessed by doctors in London. However, the publicity surrounding it has led to some suspect preparations appearing on the market. Cases of liver damage as a result of treatment with Chinese herbal teas have been reported, and unregulated preparations have occasionally been found to have been spiked with undeclared ingredients such as corticosteroids.

Loosely related to the more traditional forms of herbal medicine (and to homeopathy) are the Bach flower remedies. In 1933, a doctor called Edward Bach introduced this system of 38 flower remedies in the hope that he had found a simple method of healing. He felt that if he treated his patients' fears and anxieties and relieved them of all negative states of mind, he could free them of illness. These remedies are not commonly used for the treatment of allergies, but are widely available, have no side effects, and are unlikely to be harmful. If you do not drink alcohol for any reason, then beware: these preparations contain alcohol!

I had a bad back and had treatment from an osteopath. To my surprise, my asthma was less of a problem than usual for some time afterwards. Was this just coincidence?

It might have been coincidence, or simply being released from the stress of having a bad (and probably painful) back might have contributed to your improvement. However, some practitioners do feel that osteopathy may be useful in asthma, because it may help to improve chest movement and breathing.

Our framework of bones, muscles, ligaments and tendons supports all of our vital organs. Osteopaths base their treatment on the belief that when an injury disrupts this framework, the internal organs are affected too. Practitioners take your medical history into account before examining the way you stand and move, and testing your muscle strength. Treatment involves massage techniques, stretching, and manipulations.

Some osteopaths also practice cranial osteopathy. Although conventional medicine regards the bones which make up the skull as being rigidly fixed together, cranial osteopaths believe that they are capable of tiny movements, and that their manipulation may encourage more healthy flow of the fluid bathing the surface of the brain, thus facilitating the body's self-healing and self-balancing process. This therapy is not commonly used for allergies.

I live near a homeopathic hospital and I understand this treatment is available on the NHS. Can you tell me what homeopathic treatment involves, and would it be worth me trying it for my asthma?

The word homeopathy comes from two Greek words meaning 'similar' and 'suffering', and uses the principle of treating like with like. In homeopathy, the therapist gives minute doses of the substance which, in larger doses, would produce similar symptoms to the condition being treated. Symptoms are seen as the efforts of the body to rid itself of a particular problem, and the remedy attempts to stimulate the body to function more effectively in overcoming the disorder. In addition, remedies can be offered which aim to treat the individual's constitution in a wider sense to resolve long-standing problems. Homeopathy can take some time to show results: initially the symptoms may become worse, and it may be months before a beneficial effect is expected.

The remedies used are natural vegetable or mineral substances which are given in minute quantities. The more dilute the preparation, the more potent it is believed to be. (One of the objections to homeopathy by those who feel it has no genuine effects is that the remedies are so dilute that no trace of the original substance can actually be detected.) The remedies are safe, and side effects are rare.

As you say, homeopathy is available through the NHS, but provision is limited. There are five homeopathic hospitals in the United Kingdom (in London, Glasgow, Liverpool, Bristol and Tunbridge Wells), and some GPs are also trained in homeopathic medicine, but most practitioners work in private practice.

A number of studies have suggested that homeopathy is effective in hayfever, although none of these has been carried out in the way used to test the efficacy of conventional medicines. As hayfever is a result of the response of the body to a small number of plant proteins, it is possible to see how it might respond to treatment with related plant extracts. Eczema may also be treated homeopathically. You specifically asked about asthma, but this does not appear to respond as well to homeopathic treatments. As asthma can be brought on by a large number of triggers in any one person, this is perhaps not surprising.

I have eczema. If I was hypnotised, would it help me stop itching all the time?

In some people with eczema (and it sounds as if you may be one of them), itching can be an extremely debilitating symptom, and can have a profound effect on the quality of life. When you are hypnotised, you enter a state of very deep relaxation, during which you are more receptive to suggestions of ways of altering behaviour than you would be in a fully-conscious state. While it is most useful in reinforcing good intentions to change bad habits (eg stopping smoking), it may also be beneficial in the management of this type of itching.

I have read about enzyme potentiated desensitization (EPD). Is this something which is likely to help my allergic symptoms?

This treatment has been used by alternative allergists for the treatment of hayfever. EPD is a form of desensitization in which a mixture of allergens (including food allergens and aero-allergens) is combined with an enzyme called beta-glucuronidase, and injected in small doses under the skin. As a mixture of allergens is used, it is said there is no need to determine to which allergens you are allergic before beginning treatment.

As the dose of allergen is smaller than in conventional desensitization (discussed in the section on *Allergy explained* in Chapter 1), the risk of anaphylaxis (discussed in Chapter 6) is said to be less. However, this treatment is still potentially dangerous and should only be performed where any adverse reactions can be swiftly and properly treated. There is a study in progress evaluating the effectiveness of EPD, but as far as we can tell at present it would appear to offer no advantages over more conventional therapies.

Glossary

Terms in *italics* in these definitions refer to other terms in the glossary.

adjuvant factors Environmental factors such as air pollution and cigarette smoke which can increase an individual's risk of developing an allergic problem.

adrenal glands Important glands in the body which produce a number of hormones (chemical messengers) that are involved in the control of the body's systems.

adrenaline or **epinephrine** A natural hormone (chemical messenger) which we all have in our bodies. It is produced by the *adrenal glands* every time we exercise or are under stress or are scared, and acts on the blood vessels to maintain normal blood pressure and circulation. Adrenaline can also be administered by injection to treat the symptoms of severe allergic reactions.

aero-allergen Any *allergen* which is light enough to be carried in the air and inhaled. Examples include *dander* and *pollen*.

airway obstruction Narrowing or blockage of the passages which carry air to and from the lungs.

allergen An otherwise harmless substance which causes an allergic reaction. Once an allergy has developed, even a tiny amount of an allergen can lead to a reaction and cause allergic symptoms.

allergen immunotherapy Another name for *desensitization*.

allergic rhinitis Inflammation of the lining of the nose caused by an *allergy*. Depending on the *allergen* involved, it may be seasonal (*hayfever*) or occur all year round (*perennial allergic rhinitis*).

allergic sensitizers Another name for *sensitizers*.

allergy An abnormal or inappropriate reaction of your body's *immune*

247

system to a substance which would normally be harmless (an *allergen*).

anaphylaxis A sudden severe allergic response to an *allergen*, a potentially life-threatening reaction which involves the whole body. If untreated, it can lead to dizziness, shortness of breath, *wheezing*, palpitations, collapse and a serious drop in blood pressure. Emergency treatment is with *adrenaline* injections.

angioedema Swelling of the deep layers of the skin (the dermis) as a result of an allergic reaction. The parts of the body most commonly affected are the face and lips.

anti-inflammatory drugs Drugs which act against *inflammation*. Many diseases or conditions of the body – from *asthma* to arthritis to bowel disease – result in inflammation. Anti-inflammatory drugs reduce this inflammation and help the body to keep functioning as normal.

antibodies or **immunoglobulins** Produced by the *immune system* in response to a foreign substance, antibodies circulate in the blood and help to fight infection. They act as the immune system's memory, recognising harmful attackers such as bacteria and viruses, and assisting in their destruction.

antihistamines Drugs which block the action of *histamine*. They are used to treat allergic problems such as *hayfever* and insect stings.

asthma A condition in which *inflammation* of the airways and twitchiness of the airway wall muscles makes it difficult to move air in and out of the lungs, and causes the symptoms of *wheezing*, coughing and tightness of the chest.

atopy A tendency to develop allergic disorders such as *asthma*, *hayfever* and *eczema*. This tendency is something which is inherited genetically from your parents.

atopic dermatitis Another name for *eczema*.

biopsy The removal of a small piece of body tissue which is then examined under a microscope for diagnostic purposes.

brand name or **trade name** Most drugs have at least two names: the brand or trade name is the name given to the drug by its manufacturer, and is usually written with a capital first letter. The other name is the *generic name*. Any one drug can have several brand names but normally only one generic name.

bronchoconstriction Narrowing of the airways due to tightening of the muscles in the airway walls.

bronchodilators Drugs used in treating *asthma* which relax the muscles of the airway walls and so open up or dilate the airways. They can be taken by *inhaler* or by mouth. The medical term for *relievers*.

challenge tests or **provocation tests** Sometimes the only way to confirm an *allergy* is deliberately to provoke the symptoms it causes, using a challenge test. A small amount of a substance thought to be responsible for an allergic reaction is given in an appropriate way (eg by mouth for a food, by inhalation for an *aero-allergen*) and the resulting symptoms recorded. Challenge tests can also be used to demonstrate that a particular allergen is NOT responsible for symptoms. The tests may be *single blind* or *double blind*.

chromosome One of 46 pieces of genetic material present in all cells of the body. Each chromosome consists of a large number of *genes* carrying information inherited from our parents.

coeliac disease A disorder of the small intestine caused by an *intolerance* to *gluten*.

co-factors Additional factors which, when combined with an *allergen*, can make an allergy worse. They act as additional *triggers*.

complementary therapies Non-medical treatments which may be used in addition to conventional medical treatments. Popular complementary therapies include acupuncture, aromatherapy, homeopathy and osteopathy.

conjunctivitis *Inflammation* of the conjunctiva, which is a delicate membrane that lines the eyelids and covers the eyeball. The symptoms of conjunctivitis are itching, watering, discharge and redness of the eyes.

corticosteroids A group of chemicals produced naturally in the body by the *adrenal glands*, and which are vital for the body's own defences against infection and stress. Corticosteroids can be also be manufactured synthetically. Used as *anti-inflammatory drugs* they are powerful agents in the treatment of disorders which produce inflammation such as *asthma, eczema, hayfever, angioedema* and *anaphylaxis*.

cromoglycate or **di-sodium cromoglycate** An *anti-inflammatory drug* used in the treatment of *asthma* and *hayfever*.

Crosby capsule A small (less than 1 cm long) device used for taking a *biopsy* of the small bowel in order to diagnose *coeliac disease*.

dander Tiny particles of animal skin and the scales from their hair or fur, something like dandruff in humans. Dander is an *aero-allergen*.

decongestants Treatments which reduce swelling and congestion. Nasal decongestants are sprays or drops which relieve nasal congestion – however, as they can cause thinning and drying of the lining of the nose, they should not be used on a regular basis.

denature The permanent alteration of a protein when it is heated (or cooked) which may make it less allergenic.

depigmentation Loss of the skin's natural colour (pigment is the substance that gives skin its colour).

dermatitis An inflammatory reaction affecting the skin. In this book, used as a shorthand term for allergic contact dermatitis, caused by contact between the skin and an *allergen*. Contact may occur in a variety of ways, for example by touching the substance, swallowing a drug, or being exposed to a chemical at work.

dermatologist A doctor who specialises in the treatment of the skin and its problems and disorders.

desensitization or **immunotherapy** or **allergen immunotherapy** or **hyposensitization** A form of treatment for *allergy* in which a series of injections of very small quantities of an *allergen* are given over several months. Increasing amounts of the allergen are given in an attempt to reduce or even eliminate symptoms of the specific allergy by building up the *immune system's* tolerance to the allergen which is responsible for the problem. As this treatment is potentially dangerous, it is only available in certain circumstances in specialist centres.

dietician A person trained in nutrition who can give advice about all aspects of food and diet.

diurnal variation The change seen between one time of day and another (usually 12 hours later), in a function such as *peak expiratory flow* readings. In practical terms, this means the difference between readings taken first thing in the morning (which tend to be lower), and those taken in the evening (which tend to be higher).

double blind Describes a test (eg a *challenge test*) during which neither the doctor administering the test nor the person taking it knows whether the actual substance or a dummy substance is being given at any particular time. This means that nobody's ideas of what causes the allergic reaction can bias the results. Someone who is not involved in the testing process keeps all the records.

eczema or **atopic dermatitis** A chronic (long-lasting) inflammatory condition of the skin. In mild cases the skin is dry and scaly, but it can become red, blistered and weepy if the eczema is severe. Eczema irritates the skin and makes it itchy.

emollient A substance, usually in the form of a cream or ointment, which moisturises, softens or soothes the skin.

elimination diet or **exclusion diet** A method of confirming that a food is responsible for an allergic reaction by removing it from and then later returning it to the diet. Often different foodstuffs are tried one by one, to discover which food is causing the problem.

enteropathy Any disease of the intestine (bowel).

epinephrine The American name for *adrenaline.*

erythema Redness of the skin caused by *inflammation.*

exclusion diet Another name for an *elimination diet.*

extrinsic/intrinsic asthma An attempt to classify asthma as either being triggered by an external factor or *allergen* (ie extrinsic), or as not being associated with any obvious *allergy* (ie intrinsic). These terms are becoming less commonly used.

food diary A type of *symptom diary* which lists each and every food you have eaten and any symptoms you have had.

gastroscope A flexible tube-like viewing instrument which uses fibre optics to examine the interior of the stomach and intestines (bowels).

genes The 'units' of heredity which determine the characteristics that we inherit from our parents.

generic name Most drugs have at least two names: the generic name is the true or scientific name (usually written with a small first letter), and normally applies to all the versions of that drug, regardless of the manufacturer. The other name is the *brand name.*

gluten A protein found in wheat, oats, rye and barley which provokes an allergic response in people with *coeliac disease.*

hayfever or **seasonal allergic rhinitis** Allergic reaction to one of the *aero-allergens,* usually a plant *pollen.* Typical hayfever symptoms include a runny or stuffed-up nose, sneezing and watery eyes. They only occur during the part of the year when the pollens to which someone is allergic are being produced.

hereditary Genetically transmitted from parent to offspring.

histamine A chemical released by the cells of the body during an allergic reaction. Histamine causes *inflammation* and the symptoms of *allergy.*

hives Another name for *urticaria.*

house dust mites Microscopically tiny creatures, too small to be seen with the naked eye, which live in soft furnishings, carpets and bedding in all our houses, and which live off the human skin scales which we all shed all the time.

hymenoptera The order of insects that includes wasps and bees, which are the insects most often responsible for allergic reactions.

hyper-immunoglobulin E syndrome or **hyper-IgE syndrome** A rare condition in which vast quantities of *IgE* are made by the *immune* *system*. This leads to an exaggerated tendency towards allergic disorders, particularly *asthma* and *eczema*.

hypoallergenic 'Hypo' means 'less than' or 'lower in', so products described as hypoallergenic are lower in *allergens* than the conventional formulations. They are free from the commonest substances known to cause allergic reactions, but this does not mean that they are completely allergen-free.

hyposensitization Another name for *desensitization*.

idiopathic A description which means 'of unknown cause'. When applied to a disease or a disorder, it means that the cause of the problem is either not known or has not yet been identified.

IgE or **immunoglobulin E** The allergy *antibody*. People with allergies readily produce large amounts of IgE.

immune system The network within the body that protects us from outside 'attackers', which include viruses, bacteria and parasites, and other forms of injury.

immunoglobulins Another name for *antibodies*.

immunotherapy Another name for *desensitization*.

inflammation The body's response to injury, infection or disease. Inflammation is a reaction involving swelling, redness, tenderness or pain, itching and increased watery secretions. Generally, its purpose is to protect the body against the spread of injury or infection, but in some conditions (such as *asthma*), the inflammation becomes chronic (long-lasting), and tends to damage the body rather than protect it.

inhalers Devices used to deliver drugs so that they can be breathed in instead of being swallowed or given by injection. Inhalers are the most efficient way of giving *asthma* medications: the drugs work more quickly when inhaled (because they are delivered directly to the lungs where they are most needed) and smaller amounts are therefore needed to produce the same results.

intervention Any change made in an attempt to alter a disease process, such as reducing *house dust mite* levels.

intolerance An inability of the body adequately to handle a substance, resulting in unpleasant symptoms. For example, people who have lactose intolerance cannot digest milk properly, as they lack the body chemical (an enzyme called lactase) needed to break down lactose (the sugar in the milk). Drinking milk may give them crampy abdominal pain and diarrhoea. These symptoms are not allergic in nature, and will not occur if only tiny quantities of milk are drunk.

intradermal tests Diagnostic tests used to identify to which *allergens* someone is allergic by injecting small amounts of diluted allergen extract under the skin. A form of testing now rarely used in this country.

intrinsic asthma Discussed at the entry *extrinsic/intrinsic asthma*.

latent Temporarily concealed, ie there are no symptoms, but the disease or disorder is still present.

latex Synthetic rubber used in the manufacturer of protective gloves and similar products.

legume The pea and bean family of foods. The family includes soya bean and peanut, both of which are common causes of *allergy*.

metered dose inhaler The most common form of *inhaler* used to deliver *asthma* treatments.

multiple RAST A form of *RAST* which can test for several *allergens* at once.

nebulisers Devices which convert liquid medication into a fine mist which can then be inhaled. Nebulisers usually run on compressed air produced by an electric compressor.

nedocromil An *anti-inflammatory drug* used in the treatment of *asthma* and *hayfever*.

nettle rash Another name for *urticaria*.

occupational allergy or **workplace allergy** An *allergy* which directly results from contact with or exposure to an *allergen* found in the work environment.

over the counter medications or **OTC medications** Treatments which can be bought from pharmacists without a doctor's prescription.

passive smoking Breathing in smoke from another person's cigarette, cigar or pipe.

patch tests Diagnostic tests used to identify to which *allergens* someone is allergic, particularly useful for *dermatitis*. A small quantity of the substance to be tested is applied directly to the skin, covered, and left in place for 48 hours.

peak expiratory flow or **peak flow** A measure of how hard you can blow, ie the rate at which you can expel air from your lungs. Used to show how well your lungs are functioning, and to detect any changes in lung function.

peak flow meter A small hand-held device which measures *peak expiatory flow*.

perennial allergic rhinitis Allergic reaction to an *aero-allergen* other than *pollen*, eg to the *house dust mite* or animal *dander*. Symptoms are similar to those of *hayfever*, but occur all the year round.

pollen Small grains produced by plants as an essential part of the reproductive process. The pollen grains are the male seeds, which are light enough to be spread through the air or by insects to other plants in order to pollinate or fertilise them. Although they are too small to be seen by the naked eye, they are *allergens*, and are particularly important in *hayfever*.

pollen calendar Different plants and trees produce their flowers and their *pollens* at different times of the year, and a pollen calendar shows approximately when to expect these pollens to be released into the air.

pollen count The number of *pollen* grains found in a cubic metre of air. A count of below 50 is regarded as low, and one of over 200 as very high. *Hayfever* symptoms are usually worse when the count is high.

predisposition Susceptibility to a specific disease or disorder.

prevalence A measure of the number of people in the population with a particular medical condition at any one time. For example, if we were to say that the current prevalence of *asthma* in the UK is 10%, we would mean that 10% of the population has asthma at the moment.

preventers Drugs which are taken to prevent the symptoms of *asthma* from occurring, rather than to relieve them when they do occur. Preventers do not work immediately, but instead act over a period of time to reduce *inflammation* and stabilise the asthma. The most important preventers are the inhaled *corticosteroids*.

provocation tests Another name for *challenge tests*.

psychosomatic Relating to the influence that the mind can have on physical well-being.

PUVA Abbreviation for 'psoralen plus ultraviolet A', a treatment used for a number of skin conditions, including *eczema* and psoriasis. Psoralen is a plant extract which is taken by mouth. Two hours after taking it, the person being treated lies or sits under a machine rather like a sun lamp, which produces a type of light called ultraviolet A.

RAST or **radioallergosorbant test** A blood test which measures the amount of specific *IgE* your *immune system* has produced against a suspected *allergen*. For example, if you have *asthma*, it can confirm that you have *antibodies* against the *house dust mite*. The total amount of IgE in the blood stream is usually measured at the same time, so that the amount of any specific IgE which is found can be put into perspective.

relievers Drugs used to provide quick and effective relief from the symptoms of *asthma*. They should be used only when symptoms occur. The medical name for relievers is *bronchodilators*.

rhinitis Inflammation of the lining of the nose. *Hayfever* and *perennial allergic rhinitis* are the allergic forms of rhinitis.

rhinitis medicamentosa Chronic *rhinitis* caused by the overuse of nasal *decongestants*.

seasonal allergic rhinitis Another name for *hayfever*.

self-management plan A formal written plan, drawn up and agreed by you and your doctor, which allows you to take more responsibility for your own treatment. It sets out the circumstances in which you can take action (eg altering the dose of your medication) without first having to check with your doctor. Self-management plans often lead to an improvement in the control of an allergic disorder.

sensitizers or **allergic sensitizers** Substances which can cause allergies. This term is usually confined to substances met in the work environment which can cause *occupational allergies*.

sensitivity A reaction to a substance which is an exaggeration of a normal *side effect* produced by that substance. For example, if salbutamol (a *reliever* drug used in treating *asthma*) is given in a high enough dose, most people will develop shakiness and feel 'revved up'. People who develop these effects at a normal dose are said to be sensitive to the drug (but they are not allergic to it).

side effect Almost all drugs affect the body in ways beyond their intended actions. These unwanted 'extra' effects are called side effects. They vary in their severity from person to person, and often disappear when the body becomes used to a particular drug.

single blind Describes a test (eg a *challenge test*) in which only the doctor administering the test knows whether a real or dummy substance is being given. The person taking the test does not know which substance is which, so their ideas about what causes their symptoms cannot bias the results.

sinuses The bones of the face are not solid, but have hollow spaces within them. These spaces are the sinuses, which are joined to the air passages of the nose by small openings.

sinusitis Infection or *inflammation* of the *sinuses*. The openings of the sinuses become blocked and their drainage system disturbed. Once blocked, the pressure in the sinuses can increase because of the build-up of secretions, leading to pain which can be felt above the eyebrows, either side of the nose, or in the upper teeth.

skin prick test Diagnostic test used to identify to which *allergens* someone is allergic. A drop of a liquid preparation of the allergen is applied to the skin on the back or on the inside of the forearm, and the skin is then pricked through the droplet. The response is measured after 10-15 minutes. The procedure is painless, gives rapid results, and is probably the most commonly used and the most informative allergy test.

standardised An established measure or model to which other similar things should be compared and to which they should conform. For example, the results of a standardised test performed in one hospital should mean the same as the results of the same test carried out in a different hospital.

steroids In this book, an abbreviation for *corticosteroids*.

symptom diary A record of your symptoms and the factors thought to be causing them. People who suffer from an allergic problem are often completely well on the day on which they see their doctor, so it is therefore very useful for a doctor to see a detailed record of how serious the problem is, what form it takes, and what might be provoking it.

trade name Another name for a *brand name*.

triggers or **trigger factors** Popular name for anything which may bring on allergic symptoms or make them worse. For example, triggers for *asthma* include exercise, emotion, changes in air temperature and air pollution.

urticaria or **nettle rash** or **hives** Swelling of the superficial layers of the skin, usually as a result of an allergic reaction. The characteristic itchy lumps (called weals or hives) last for only a few hours.

weal A bump in the skin produced as a response to an *allergen*.

wheeze or **wheezing** A high-pitched noise produced when breathing out. It comes from the chest and not the throat.

workplace allergy Another name for an *occupational allergy*.

Appendix 1

Diagnosing your allergies

In this appendix my aim has been to give you a description of each of the common allergy tests, including details of what you will feel and whether or not they are uncomfortable. I have also suggested when each test may be needed, pointed out any special instructions relating to the tests, and discussed their individual advantages and disadvantages. I hope this information will help you to understand why your doctor has chosen one test rather than another. I have also briefly described a number of tests sometimes used by alternative practitioners, although few of these are felt to have a place in the diagnosis of allergy.

Why test?

If you have suffered an allergic reaction and its cause is uncertain or unknown, you will need to have one or more of the tests described here. Even if you know the cause of your allergic reaction, you may still need to have the diagnosis confirmed by some form of allergy testing, particularly if you have had a severe allergic reaction, or if you have multiple allergies, or if your doctor is considering any form of treatment which is going to be long-lasting, difficult, time-consuming or expensive. If you are going to help with the evaluation of a new treatment, you will certainly need to have your allergy confirmed by formal testing. If there is any confusion as to whether your problem is caused by a true allergy (that is, one involving the production of the allergy antibody IgE, as discussed in the section on *Allergy explained* in Chapter 1) or whether some other process is involved, allergy testing can clear up this doubt. Finally, if having an allergy has any legal implications for you (for example, if you might be eligible for compensation), then the diagnosis must be confirmed by appropriate tests.

Each year 10% of the population of the United Kingdom experience an allergic problem of some kind, and 25% of the population will, during their lifetimes, see a doctor because of an allergy. As these problems are now so common, allergy testing is being carried out more often and is becoming increasingly sophisticated. However, there is no point in doing allergy tests if either you or your doctor are going to be unwilling to take action based on the results. If a true allergy is diagnosed, you may benefit not only from medications aimed at treating the allergic reaction once it has happened, but also from preventive action, both in the form of drugs and in the form of allergen avoidance.

Choosing the most suitable test

Different allergies are more common at different ages, and so the type of allergy test you will be offered by your doctor depends, to some extent, on your age. Food allergies are more common in infancy and early childhood, whereas problems caused by allergens in the air become more common after the age of 5 years. Allergies to insect stings usually start in adulthood, and can be particularly troublesome in the elderly.

Every test performed in the diagnosis of allergies should be:

- relevant (there is no point in doing skin prick testing or patch testing unless you include the likely culprits);
- standardised (so that the result of a test done in one hospital means the same as that done in a different hospital);
- repeatable (so that the results on one occasion can be compared with the results of the same test on a different occasion);
- specific (so that the test is only positive in people who have that allergy); and
- sensitive (so that the test is only negative in people who do not have the problem).

This is a lot to ask of any test, and it is impossible for any one test to score 100% on all of these points. Every test has its advantages and its disadvantages, and this is why specialist knowledge is necessary to make sure that the right test is chosen for you.

By far the most useful information available to your doctor will come from your medical history – the account that you give of your allergic reaction and your answers to a large number of questions, including the following:

- your general status (age, job, and so on);
- any illnesses you have had in the past;
- whether there are other members of your family with allergic problems;
- the details of your own allergic problems; and
- how often you are exposed to allergens and to other factors which can make allergic problems worse, eg cigarette smoke, air pollution and certain drugs.

All of these details must be taken into account when assessing the result of any allergy test. If your allergy is particularly troublesome or if you have had a severe allergic reaction, it is advisable that you be referred to an allergy specialist.

Skin prick testing

Description
This is probably the most commonly used allergy test. It is performed on the skin of your back or of your inner forearm (as shown in Figure 14), and you can be tested to up to 25 allergens at any one time. A drop of the allergen extract is placed on your skin, which is pricked through the drop using a lancet (a small sharp prong just 1 mm long). A positive result consists of a weal (a pale bump) which may be itchy and surrounded by a red area or flare. The size of the weal is measured after 10 minutes, and any weal of greater than 2 mm (or, in some cases, 3 mm) in size is regarded as being positive.

Two additional substances will always be included in this form of testing: a positive and a negative control. The positive control solution contains histamine, to which everyone should react. Failure to do so can result from treatment with certain medicines (including antihistamines, corticosteroids, and certain antidepressant drugs) and will alert the tester to the fact that the results of testing will be unreliable. The negative control is made from a saline solution, to which

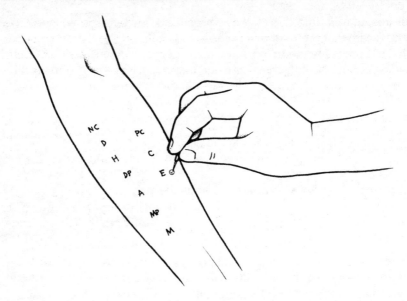

Figure 14: Skin prick testing on the skin of the inner forearm.

no one should react. A positive reaction to this negative control shows that the skin is, for some reason, extremely sensitive, and once again indicates that testing will not be reliable.

Skin prick testing is a painless procedure, which is well tolerated even by small infants. Positive reactions may be somewhat itchy, but this will subside within an hour.

Skin prick testing is a very sensitive diagnostic tool, and not everyone who has a positive test has symptoms of an allergy. If you do not develop a reaction to an allergen, you can be almost certain that you are not allergic to it. However, a positive reaction may be highlighting a hidden or latent allergy which is not currently causing you problems, but which might show up later on in your life.

Indications
Skin prick testing is usually the first test recommended when an allergy is suspected.

Special instructions
Tell the person doing the skin prick testing if you are on any medication.

If it is safe to do so, treatment with antihistamines, corticosteroids or tricyclic antidepressants should be stopped for an appropriate time (up to two weeks) before the test is carried out. However, these medications should only be stopped on your doctor's instructions.

Advantages
This is a simple, quick and inexpensive form of testing, which can be performed to a very wide range of different allergens. It can give useful information in all forms of allergy, and provides results within 15 minutes.

Disadvantages
Skin prick testing is unreliable in the very young and the elderly. It cannot be performed if you are taking certain medications (listed earlier in this section) or in people with severe eczema. Although generally extremely safe, skin prick testing may provoke a severe allergic reaction in people who have previously experienced anaphylaxis (discussed in Chapter 6), although this is extremely rare.

Intradermal testing

Description
Intradermal literally means 'within the skin', from the Latin word 'intra' meaning 'within' and the Greek word 'derma' meaning 'skin'. In this test a small amount of a diluted allergen extract is injected beneath the surface of your skin. A reaction is usually apparent within 10-20 minutes, and takes the form of swelling, itching and a raised weal (a pale bump).

This form of testing is now rarely used in this country, as not only does it give inaccurate results (using a high concentration of allergen can falsely indicate allergy where none exists) but also it can be dangerous, with a higher risk of anaphylactic reactions (anaphylaxis is discussed in Chapter 6).

Patch testing

Description
For this test allergens are prepared in appropriate concentrations in

white soft paraffin (eg Vaseline) and are then spread on to discs the size of a one pence piece. The discs (which are made of a special metal which cannot itself provoke a reaction) are placed on your skin (usually on your back, as shown in Figure 15) and covered with an adhesive dressing. They are left in place for 48 hours, after which your skin is examined, and any redness and swelling are noted. Your skin will be re-examined after a further 48 hours for any remaining redness or swelling. The interpretation of this form of testing is not as simple as it sounds, and should only be done by someone with skill and experience.

Indications
Patch testing is performed in cases of contact dermatitis where allergy is suspected.

Special instructions
The symptoms of contact dermatitis must be brought under control using an appropriate steroid cream before patch testing can be carried out, or else the results will be unreliable. These steroid creams should

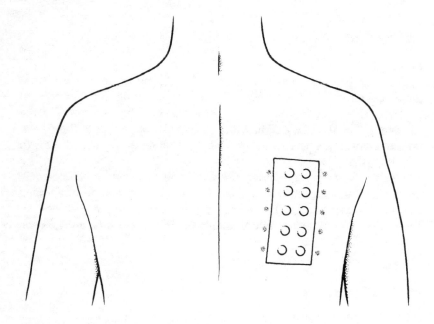

Figure 15: Patch testing on the skin of the back.

then be discontinued for at least 3-4 weeks before testing, as they may suppress the test response.

Advantages
This is a relatively simple, safe and inexpensive form of testing, which is particularly useful for all forms of contact dermatitis.

Disadvantages
Interpretation of the results is not easy, and requires a thorough knowledge of your allergy history and of the materials in question. Almost 10% of the normal healthy population with no skin disease will demonstrate unexpected, apparently irrelevant, positive results. Itching or blistering may develop as a response to the test allergens.

Radioallergosorbant test (RAST)

Description
This is a blood test which measures the amount of specific IgE your immune system has produced against a suspected allergen. For example, if you have asthma, it can confirm that you have antibodies against the house dust mite. (There is more information about IgE and other antibodies in the section on *Allergy explained* in Chapter 1.)

The test is carried out on a small sample of blood which is taken from a vein in your arm, using a fine needle and a small syringe. Although some people dislike needles, the blood test causes minimal discomfort. The sample is then sent to a specialist laboratory, and the results are available within a few days.

RAST uses a technique in which a radioactive label is allowed to attach itself to the IgE present in your blood sample. Measuring the amount of radioactivity left at the completion of the test provides information about any specific antibodies you have produced. The total amount of IgE in your blood stream is usually measured at the same time, so that the amount of any specific IgE which is found can be compared to the total amount in your blood.

Indications
This test is increasing in popularity, and is often used in conjunction with skin prick testing. It is particularly useful when the risk of an anaphylactic reaction (discussed in Chapter 6) makes skin prick testing

too risky; when extensive eczema makes skin prick testing impractical; and when allergic symptoms are so severe that antihistamine medication cannot be discontinued to permit accurate skin prick testing.

Special instructions
Local anaesthetic cream may be available for small children and for adults who particularly request it, to eliminate any discomfort from blood sampling. This cream takes an hour to be effective, so must be applied and covered by an adhesive dressing in advance of the test.

Advantages
This form of allergy testing is completely safe. It is specific, in that if a RAST is positive it is likely that you have a true allergy, but false negative results can occur.

Disadvantages
The test involves taking a sample of blood, which some people find unpleasant. It is expensive. A negative result does not completely rule out the possibility that allergy to that allergen exists. Do not assume that you are not at risk from a particular allergen just because the RAST is negative.

Other blood tests

Multiple RAST

A form of RAST which can test for several allergens at once is now available, and is being marketed commercially through a number of large supermarkets. Because this form of testing can yield positive results when no allergy is present (false positives), as well as giving negative results when an allergy does in fact exist (false negatives), it should not be performed without the results being put in the context of a full medical history and interpreted by a trained doctor.

Other antibody tests

Although most allergy testing involves looking for evidence of the IgE antibody, in some circumstances (such as coeliac disease, discussed in Chapter 5) evidence of other antibodies such as IgA or IgG is helpful in making a diagnosis. (There is more information about these antibodies in the section on *Allergy explained* in Chapter 1.) As far as you are concerned, the test simply involves giving a blood sample as you would for RAST (as described in the previous section of this appendix).

Challenge tests

Sometimes the only way to confirm an allergy is deliberately to provoke the symptoms it causes. Challenge tests (also called provocation tests) can also be used to demonstrate that a particular allergen is NOT responsible for your symptoms.

Airways challenge tests

Description
You inhale increasing concentrations of either a histamine-like substance or of a specific allergen solution made from the substance suspected of causing your asthma or hayfever symptoms. Your response to each dose is measured using lung function tests (described later in this appendix). The test is continued until there is a predetermined drop in your lung function. At this point, your chest may feel a little tight and you may be a little wheezy, but these symptoms will be mild. Your lung function is then returned to normal by giving you a bronchodilator (reliever) inhaler to use (these inhalers are discussed in the section on *Treatment* in Chapter 2).

Indications
This form of testing is rarely used, but it can be particularly useful in the diagnosis of asthma brought on by substances encountered in the workplace. It is also used in allergy research.

Special instructions
Bronchodilator medications and drinks containing caffeine must be avoided for at least four hours before testing, and you must be free from colds.

Advantages
This form of testing can be very useful when it is helpful for your doctor to have a measurable or quantifiable response, for example to find out if one drug suits you better than another, or to see if someone's asthma gets better when he or she stops working with a particular chemical.

Disadvantages
Although it is not painful, this procedure can be rather intimidating because of the equipment used, and requires a high degree of co-operation from the person being tested. Because of this, it cannot usually be performed on children under 7 years old. If an allergen is used, you will be kept under observation for at least eight hours after the test. There is a small risk of a severe asthma reaction, so this form of testing will only be performed by an experienced practitioner who has the facilities available to handle emergencies. These tests are relatively time-consuming and therefore expensive.

Oral challenge tests (food challenges)

Description
The food or foods suspected of causing allergic reactions are eliminated completely from your diet. If your symptoms disappear, these foods are reintroduced one at a time, at intervals of at least three days, to see if your symptoms recur. To make sure that your ideas on what causes your symptoms cannot bias the results, foods are often reintroduced in capsule form so that you don't know which food is which (this is called a single blind challenge). Even better is the form of challenge in which neither you nor your doctor knows which food is being reintroduced (a double blind challenge). In a double blind challenge, someone who is not involved with the testing process keeps the records.

Indications
This form of testing can be useful when food allergy has been previously diagnosed using inappropriate or invalid tests; when your symptoms are not typical of an allergy but may be due to some form of food intolerance; or when several skin prick test results are positive and it is unclear which of the foods tested is causing your symptoms.

Special instructions
This form of testing should never be performed on anyone who has suffered an anaphylactic reaction due to food allergy (anaphylaxis is discussed in Chapter 6).

Advantages
Double blind food challenge is extremely reliable, and if an allergy is present, symptoms will appear when the food responsible is introduced. If no symptoms occur, allergy can be ruled out.

Disadvantages
There is a risk of severe allergic or anaphylactic reactions, so this form of testing should only be carried out in a hospital by expert and experienced medical staff who are fully trained and equipped to handle emergencies.

Lung function testing

Two forms of lung function test are commonly used in the diagnosis of asthma, both of which simply involve you blowing out air as hard and as fast as you can into the mouthpiece of a piece of equipment. Full lung spirometry (which measures how quickly and efficiently you can empty your lungs) is generally only carried out in a hospital, as the equipment required is relatively expensive, although some GPs now have this facility. Peak expiratory flow testing, which is described here, is more commonly used as you can do it at home.

Peak expiratory flow testing

Description
This test is also known as peak flow testing or peak flow monitoring. It uses a peak expiratory flow meter (more usually called a peak flow meter), which is a small hand-held device that measures how fast air can be blown out from your lungs. If you have asthma, not only will your readings be lower than those of people without asthma who are of your age, height and gender (all things which affect the readings), but your readings will also be more variable from day to day. One-off readings are therefore not particularly helpful, so you will usually be given your own meter and asked to keep twice-daily recordings on a special chart, recording the best of three readings each time.

To make a reading, you take a full deep breath in, you place the instrument between your lips so that an airtight seal is made between your lips and the mouthpiece, and you then blow through the device as hard and as fast as you can. Air passing through the meter moves a small pointer across a scale, indicating the maximum flow achieved. The pointer must be reset before each blow.

Indications
Peak flow recordings can be useful in the following situations:

- to diagnose asthma;

- to judge whether or not a particular treatment is leading to improvement;
- to help judge the need for increased treatment if your asthma is going out of control;
- if you find it difficult to judge how bad your asthma is;
- in asthma research.

Special instructions
You should have your own device, as readings can vary slightly between meters. The device should be cleaned regularly according to the manufacturer's instructions. You should be taught how to use the meter correctly, and your technique should be reviewed regularly by your doctor or practice nurse.

Advantages
Peak flow meters are relatively inexpensive, and can provide information which can be extremely helpful in the day-to-day management of asthma. For example, you and your doctor can agree on a self-management plan, which will allow you to use your peak flow readings to judge the amount of treatment you require, and to take steps to deal with any changes in your symptoms without the need to call for medical help each time.

Disadvantages
Peak flow recordings should not be used as the sole indicator of how good or bad your lungs are on any particular day – the meters are not infallible, so you should also take note of how your chest feels and what symptoms you are experiencing. It is possible to cheat with a peak flow meter, producing both falsely high and falsely low recordings.

Symptom diaries

Description
Your doctor may ask you to keep a record of both your symptoms and of the factors thought to be causing them, for example a record of your bowel symptoms together with a list of all the foods you have eaten. Sometimes special forms are provided, but an ordinary notebook will do.

Indications
A symptom diary can be an invaluable source of information in almost any allergic problem.

Special instructions
Your doctor will explain to you exactly what is required, but you should feel free to include any extra information which you think might be helpful.

Advantages
People who suffer from allergic problems are often completely well on the days on which they see their doctors. It is therefore extremely useful to be able to take with you a record of how frequent and how serious your problem is, what form it takes, and what might be provoking it.

Disadvantages
Not only is a symptom diary subjective, it also requires you – if it is to be of any use – to be totally honest and comprehensive when recording your exposure to allergens and any possible resulting symptoms. It may take many weeks to record enough details to provide useful information and this can require considerable effort on your part. Symptom diaries can also be difficult to interpret.

Bowel biopsy

Description
In order to diagnose coeliac disease, a bowel biopsy is necessary, and there are two ways in which this can be done. The method chosen will depend upon which technique is preferred at the hospital you attend. Both methods provide a small piece of bowel lining which can then be examined under a microscope.

The first method uses an instrument called a gastroscope, which is a flexible tube-like viewing instrument that uses fibre optics to allow the doctor to see the inside of your digestive system. The gastroscope is inserted into your stomach or small intestine through your mouth, and a small amount of the bowel lining is taken once the instrument is in the correct position. This technique is generally used in adults.

The second method involves a small (less than 1 cm long) capsule called a Crosby capsule, which is attached to a very fine hollow tube. Again this is passed into the intestine via the mouth. Once it is in the correct position (confirmed by an X-ray), the capsule is triggered to take a small amount of the bowel lining, and then gently withdrawn. This technique is more commonly used in children.

Although both these procedures sound rather unpleasant, they are not actually as disagreeable as they appear. They are usually tolerated well, even by very small children. You will be given a sedative to help you relax while the test is being carried out. It is essential that coeliac disease is diagnosed accurately using one of these biopsy techniques, as the treatment involves lifelong avoidance of all foods containing gluten. This strict diet is not something that you would want to have to follow unnecessarily.

Environmental testing

This is a test on your surroundings, not on you. A number of substances found in the environment – both at home and at work – can cause allergic problems. Occasionally it is helpful to send samples of dust, air or chemical substances used at work for analysis. This type of testing can only be done by a specialist allergy centre.

Other tests

Alternative allergy specialists often use diagnostic tests other than the ones I have described above, and these can include the following.

Applied kinesiology

This measures muscle strength before and after exposure to a suspected allergen.

Auricular cardiac reflex method

Close proximity to a substance to which a person is allergic is said to result in a change in position in the strongest pulse at the wrist.

Hair analysis

The subject's hair is examined and medical problems are diagnosed from the appearance and content of the hair.

Leukocytotoxic tests

White blood cells are put into contact with the suspected allergen and the cells are observed under a microscope for changes in size and shape. These changes are regarded as an indication of the cells' reactivity.

Neutralisation-provocation testing (the Miller technique)

The dose of an allergen which can switch off or neutralise the allergy is found, and this dose is administered as drops under the subject's tongue.

Vega testing

This measures the electromagnetic fields produced by the subject, using a Vegatest machine.

These tests are not felt by conventional medical practitioners to be relevant, standardised or repeatable, and are considered to have no place in the diagnosis of true allergy.

Appendix 2

Useful addresses

Allergy associations, organisations and self-help groups

Anaphylaxis Campaign
The Ridges
2 Clockhouse Road
Farnborough
Hampshire GU14 7QY
Tel: 01252 542029 (01252 318723
   after office hours)

Asthma Society of Ireland
Eden House
15–17 Eden Quay
Dublin 1, Ireland
Tel: 00 353 1 878 8511

British Allergy Foundation
Deepdene House
30 Bellegrove Road
Welling
Kent DA16 3PY
Tel: 0181 303 8525
Helpline tel: 0891 516500
   (9.00 am-5.00 pm Mon-Fri)

Coeliac Society
PO Box 220
High Wycombe
Buckinghamshire HP11 2HY
Tel: 01494 437278

National Asthma Campaign
Providence House
Providence Place
London N1 0NT
Tel: 0171 226 2260
Helpline tel: 0345 010203 (9.00
   am-7.00 pm Mon-Fri, calls
   charged at local rate)

National Asthma and Respiratory
   Training Centre
The Athanaeum
10 Church Street
Warwick CV34 4AB
Tel: 01926 493313

National Eczema Society
163 Eversholt Street
London NW1 IBU
Tel: 0171 388 4097

Equipment manufacturers and suppliers

Clement Clarke Ltd
Edinburgh Way
Harlow
Essex CM20 2TT
Tel: 01279 414969
Peak flow meters

Dunlopillo Ltd
Station Road
Pannal
Harrogate
North Yorkshire HG3 1JL
Tel: 01423 872411
Latex foam mattresses and
    pillows

Medic-Aid Ltd
Heath Place
Bognor Regis
West Sussex PO22 9SL
Tel: 01243 840888
Nebulisers, compressors, face
    masks and spacer devices

Vitalograph Ltd
Maids Moreton House
Buckingham MK18 1SW
Tel: 01280 822811
Peak flow meters

Identification jewellery

Golden Key
1 Hare Street
Sheerness
Kent ME12 1AH
Tel: 01795 663403

Medic-Alert Foundation
1 Bridge Wharf
156 Caledonian Road
London N1 9BR
Tel: 0171 833 3034

SOS Talisman
Talman Ltd
21 Grays Corner
Ley Street
Ilford
Essex IG2 7RQ
Tel: 0181 554 5579

Pollen count and air pollution information

Daily Pollen Update (in season only)
Different number every year: check with National Asthma Campaign (Tel: 0171 226 2260) each spring

Department of the Environment Pollution Helpline
Tel: 0800 556677 (calls are free)
Recorded message giving air quality information including a forecast of pollution levels

Pollen Enquiries
Pollen Research Unit
National Pollution Network
University College Worcester
Henwick Grove
Worcester WR2 6AJ
Send s.a.e. and allow 3 weeks for reply
Website:
http://pollenuk.worc.ac.uk

Other useful addresses

ASH (Action on Smoking and Health)
16 Fitzhardinge Street
London W1H 9PL
Tel: 0171 224 0743

Department for Education and Employment (DFEE)
Publications Centre
PO Box 6927
London E3 3NZ
Tel: 0845 602226

Department of Health
Richmond House
79 Whitehall
London SW1A 2NF
Tel: 0171 210 4850
Health literature line tel: 0800 555 777 (calls are free)

Foresight
28 The Paddock
Godalming
Surrey GU7 1XD
Tel: 01483 427839
Advice and counselling on preconceptual care

Health and Safety Executive
Information Centre
Broad Lane
Sheffield S3 7HQ
Tel: 0114 289 2345
Book orders: 01787 881165

Health Education Authority
Hamilton House
Mabledon Place
London WC1H 9TX
Tel: 0171 383 3833

Holiday Care Service
2nd Floor
Imperial Buildings
Victoria Road
Horley
Surrey RH6 7PZ
Tel: 0129 377 4535
Holiday advice for people with
  special needs, including
  information on transport,
  insurance, oxygen supplies, etc.

Institute of Translation and
  Interpreting
377 City Road
London EC1V 1NA
Tel: 0171 713 7600

Ministry of Agriculture, Fisheries
  and Food (MAFF)
MAFF Publications
London SE99 7TP
Tel: 0645 556 000 (calls charged at
  local rate)
Booklets on food labelling, food
  additives, nutrition and food
  safety

Ministry of Agriculture, Fisheries
  and Food (MAFF)
MAFF Consumer Helpline
Room 306C
Ergon House
c/o Nobel House
17 Smith Square
London SW1P 3JR
Tel: 0345 573012 (calls charged at
  local rate)
Factsheets on food allergies and
  intolerance

Quit (National Society for Non-
  smokers)
Victory House
170 Tottenham Court Road
London W1P 0HA
Tel: 0171 388 5775
Quitline (telephone helpline):
  0800 002200 (calls are free)

Appendix 3

Useful publications

At the time of writing, all the publications listed here were available. When a title has been mentioned in this book, it is marked with an asterisk (*).

I have indicated the titles which are available free of charge; for all other items we suggest you check current prices with your local bookshop or with the publishers. Your local library may have copies of some of the books mentioned, either for loan or as reference copies.

In addition to the publications listed here, the various allergy associations, organisations and self-help groups publish a wide range of magazines, booklets, leaflets and factsheets. Contact them at the addresses given in Appendix 2 for up-to-date publications lists.

Asthma

Asthma at Your Fingertips, by Mark Levy, Sean Hilton and Greta Barnes, published by Class Publishing (second edition 1997)

The Asthma Handbook, by Jenny Lewis with the National Asthma Campaign, published by Vermilion (1996)

Living with Asthma and Hayfever, by John Donaldson, published by Penguin (revised edition 1994)

*If you have asthma because of your work (leaflet NI 237), issued by the Department of Social Security, and available on request from local Social Security offices

Skin allergies

Eczema in Childhood – the Facts, by David J.Atherton, published by Oxford University Press (revised edition 1995)

The Eczema Handbook, by Jenny Lewis with the National Eczema Society, published by Vermilion (1994)

Hayfever

*Hayfever in the Garden, published by Hoechst Marion Roussel (copies available free from Hoechst Marion Roussel, Broadwater Park, North Orbital Road, Denham, Uxbridge, Middx UB9 5HP. Tel: 01895 834343)

Living with Asthma and Hayfever, by John Donaldson, published by Penguin (revised edition 1994)

Anaphylaxis

Life-threatening Allergic Reactions, by Dr Deryk Williams, Anna Williams and Laura Croker, published by Piatkus Books (1997)

General and miscellaneous

Allergies A-Z by Myron Lipkowitz, published by Facts on File (1994)

*HEA Guide to Complementary Medicine and Therapies by Anne Woodham, published by the Health Education Authority (1994)

Living Allergy Free by M. Eric Gershwin, published by Humana Press (1992)

*Patient's Charter, published by the Department of Health (single copies available free of charge by calling 0800 555 777)

*Patient's Charter Services for Children and Young People (the full title of the booklet popularly known as the Children's Charter), published by the Department of Health (single copies available free of charge by calling 0800 555 777)

*Special Educational Needs – A Guide for Parents, published by the Department for Education and Employment (single copies available free from the DFEE Publications Centre)

*Supporting Pupils with Medical Needs in Schools, published by the Department for Education and Employment (single copies available free from the DFEE Publications Centre)

*Traveller's Guide to Health, published by the Department of Health (single copies available free of charge by calling 0800 555 777)

Index

NOTE: Page references in *italic* refer to illustrations.

abdominal discomfort or pain 8,
16, 123, 132, 155
acne 112–13
antibiotic for 112
action plan for living with
anaphylaxis 167
acupuncture 114, 240–2
see also shiatsu
acyclovir 86
addiction to inhalers 48
additives
food 58
washing powder 78
adhesives 91
adjuvant factors (increasing risk)
20, 27, 247
admission to hospital *see* hospital
adrenal glands 247
adrenaline 145, 154, 158–9, *159*,
247
by inhaler 160
importance of carrying it at all
times 157–8, *159*, 160–1, 198
injection of 158–61, 165, 167,
195, 198
adults and children, difference in
asthma treatments 49–50
aero-allergens 94, 220, 247

Aerobec 52
Aerolin 8, 38, 49, 52
age
and allergy 10, 20, 28
and asthma 29, 55
and hayfever 95, 179
and reaction to antibiotics 63
air
air conditioning 183
cold 20, 32
in lungs *see* peak flow meter
national quality standards 103
pollens carried by 103
pollution 29, 95, 103–4
in asthma 33, 35, 59–60
chemical 20, 27
quality reports 105, 232
temperature 34, 57
air travel *see* flying
airways
challenge tests 265–6
narrowing of 13, 25, 35, 38
swelling and obstruction 153,
247
alcohol
and antihistamines 117–18
in Bach flower remedies 244
in bath oils 73, 78

279

alcohol *(continued)*
    and digestion 122
    and drowsiness 108, 116
allergen avoidance 55, 217–38
    in general 216–20, 247
allergen desensitization *see*
    desensitization
allergen immunotherapy *see*
    desensitization
allergens
    and asthma 32, 55
    causing anaphylactic reactions
        162
    description of 16–17, 247
    food 235–8
    in hospital 208
allergic conjunctivitis 9
allergic contact dermatitis *see*
    dermatitis
allergic rhinitis *see* rhinitis
allergic shiners 97
allergy 14
    and asthma 55–60
    at work *see* work, allergies at
    cure 11
    description of 4, 247–8
    developing over many years 88,
        92
    food 33
        see also individual foods
    and holidays 190–1
    how it happens 6–7
    or intolerance 7–8
    knowing if you are allergic
        14–15
    living with 188–216
    parts of body affected 9
    preventing children from
        developing 219–20
    in schoolchildren 22
    seasonal 11

allergy *(continued)*
    why some and not others 18
    symptoms 6
    to animals *see* animals
    to antibiotics 63–4
        see also antibiotics;
        individual allergies
    true 8, 16
allergy testing service in
    supermarket 142
almonds 133
alstroemeria 181
alternative remedies 144
    see also complementary
        remedies
altitude
    and allergens 219
    and house dust mites 219, 222
aluminium 37
ambulance in emergency 158, 160,
    167
    abroad 191
    see also emergency treatment
Ambulance Service 36
amicillin, Amoxil, amoxycillin 64,
    171
anabolic steroids 49, 53, 76
anaesthetics
    fear of anaphylaxis while under
        207–8
    general 205–6
anaphylactic shock 129, 145, 152
    knowing you are at risk 155–6
anaphylaxis 9, 11, 23, 130, 151–71
    and admission to hospital 207
    and adrenaline injection 161
    explanation 152–3, 248
    food-dependent exercise-
        induced 166
    identifying cause 162–6
    idiopathic 165

anaphylaxis *(continued)*
  inability to diagnose 165
  living with 166–71
  symptoms 153–4
Anaphylaxis Campaign 129, 195
angioedema 9, 23, 63, 248
  in food allergies 130, 155
animals 17, 27, 34, 35, 37, 56, 60
  and bedding 223–4
  cosmetic testing 89–90
  and hayfever 94
  how they produce allergens 233
  non-allergenic 235
  pet allergens 232–5
  working with 186–7
  see also individual animals
ankles, eczema of 66
anti-allergy covers for bedding
  225
anti-house dust mite sprays 18
anti-inflammatory drugs 33, 63–4,
  247
antibiotics
  for acne 112
  allergy to 63–5
  for eczema 79
  in hayfever 101
  side effects 101
antibodies 5, 248
  allergy 4, 6
antihistamine 49, 55–6, 57, 68,
  107, 248
  after bee or wasp stings 162
  and alcohol 117–18
  combined with antibiotics
    112–13
  and driving safely 116
  non-sedating type 113, 116
  sleepiness while taking 108
  tablets 107, 110–11, 160
antioxidant in food 58

antiseptic creams 133
antiseptics 91
anxiety *see* stress
applied kinesiology test 270
apricots 136
arachis 166
armed services, working in 36
aromatherapy 242–3
arthritis
  and urticaria 62
  and use of inhalers 50
ascorbic acid 63
aspirin 20, 33, 62, 64, 74
  after bee or wasp stings 162
  gargle with 100
  under-twelves 100
astemizole 108, 117
asthma 4, 9, 12, 24–54, 248
  acupuncture 241–2
  acute attack 31, 43, 48
  age 29, 55
  allergy 55–60
  animals 34, 35
  aromatherapy 242
  causes of 26–8
  control of 28, 40, 48, 51, 53
  cure 29–30
  desensitization for 11, 54
  diagnosis and assessment
    37–42
  dosage of preventer inhaler
    50–1
  in early childhood 20
  and eczema 68, 72
  environment 29
  exercise 34–5
  explanation 25–30
  flying 193
  food allergies 130
  forestry work 181–2
  general anaesthetic 205

asthma *(continued)*
  general health 35
  and hayfever 68, 95
  history of 24–5
  hobbies 34
  holidays 190
  homeopathy 245–6
  and house dust mites 19, 222
  incidence of *21*, 23
  increased severity of symptoms 36
  non-seasonal 11
  occupational 36–7, 173, 174, 175–6
  osteopathy teatment 244–5
  and pregnancy *see* pregnancy
  reliever inhalers for 8
  school trips 203
  seasonal 57
  side-effects of treatments 51–3
  special schooling 204–5
  sport 34–5
  stabilisation of 43
  starting school 196–7
  stress 19
  symptoms 25, 30–2
  triggers 32–7, 49, 54, 55
  typical symptoms 30
  uniqueness of symptoms 30, 39
  variation in severity 28, 176
  weather 34, 57
asthma clinic 44
atopic dermatitis *see* dermatitis
atopy 4–5, 6, 10, 14, 17, 18, 248
  animals 232
  asthma 26
  food allergies 126–7
  skin allergies 62, 66, 68–9
  see also inheritance
Atrovent 49, 52
Augmentin 171

auricular cardiac reflex test 270
Autohaler 45–6, *46*
avoiding allergens 55, 217–38
azlocillin 171

babies
  born during pollen season 20, 27
  breast-feeding 58
  eczema 66, 68–9
  exposure to allergens 27, 70
  food allergies 126
  maternal smoking 20, 27
  spacer devices for 49
  tobacco smoke 220
  vaccination against allergy 11
  weaning 126
Bach flower remedies 244
bacteria 5
bananas 134, 237
barley 134, 136, 150
barrier covers against house dust mites 224–5
barrier creams 179
bath oil for eczema 72, 73, 74, 77–8
baths and eczema 73
batter 238
beans 62, 136
beclomethasone 52
Beconase Hayfever nasal spray 107
Becotide 52, 53
bedrooms *see* beds and bedding
beds and bedding 18, 70–1, 86, 200, 222–6
  in hospital 207
bee stings 11, 12, 62
  anaphylactic reactions 153, 154, 155, 162, 168–9
  avoiding being stung 168–9, 170

bee stings *(continued)*
  desensitization 169–70
  how to remove 162
beef 137
benzene 104
beta-blocker drugs 33
beta-glucuronidase 246
biscuits 238
black-eyed peas 136
blackberries 136
blankets 224
bleeding, nose 99
blisters 84, 86
blood pressure
  high 33
  serious drop in 130, 155, 158
blood tests 38, 149, 163, 263–5
blood vessels, enlargement of 95
bloodshot eyes 102
bloodstream, rapid spread of
  anaphylactic reaction 155
blueness in bad asthma attacks 31
blurred vision 52
bone strength in children 49
boots, rubber 87
Boots Medilink service 171
bottle-feeding 58
bowel biopsy for coeliac disease
  149, 248, 269–70
bowel problems
  and allergy 7, 9, 13, 14, 80
  and food allergies 122, 123
  occupational 174
brand names for drugs 192, 248
brazil nuts 136
bread 238
breast-feeding 58
  asthma treatment during 211–12
  and food allergies 126, 127
  hayfever medications during
    107, 211–12

breast-feeding *(continued)*
  and proteins 70
breath-actuated dry powder
  device *see* Diskhaler;
  Turbohaler
breath-actuated metered dose
  inhaler *see* Autohaler
breathing
  in asthma 25–6
  difficulties in 9, 187
  through mouth in hayfever 100
breathlessness
  in anaphylaxis 130, 131
  in asthma attack 31
Bricanyl 52
British Allergy Foundation 195,
  197, 216, 223
British Society for Allergy and
  Clinical Immunology 170
bronchi *see* airways
bronchodilator drugs 38, 49, 248
Brufen 33, 62, 64
bubble baths 72, 73
buckles (containing nickel) 90
budesonide 52
buildings 183
bulbs, flower 87, 181
bullying at school affecting
  eczema 202
butter 238

cake 238
calcium, source of 81, 82
canned food 58
capsules, in food challenge
  testing 140
car
  bees or wasps trapped inside
    169
  suitable type for hayfever
    sufferers 116, 231

car *(continued)*
 see also driving safely
carbon monoxide 104
carpets 222, 223, 224
carrots 134
casein and caseinates 238
cashew nuts 136
castor oil plants 17
catarrh 101
catering work and eczema 183–4
cats 13, 27, 35, 56–7, 69, 78, 106,
 232–4
 and childhood eczema 86–7
cells, of immune system 14
central heating 18, 29, 60, 69,
 227–8
cereals 238
cetirizine 12, 68, 108, 118
CFCs in asthma inhalers 53–4,
 108
challenge tests 122, 131, 140,
 163–4
 airways 265–6
 description 249, 265
 oral 266
cheese 85, 123, 126, 238
Chelsea Flower Show, low
 allergen garden 231
chemical, reaction to 7
chemical messengers (hormones)
 14, 158
chemicals 9, 67, 73
 and asthma 29, 36
 and dermatitis 87–9, 179, 185–6
 and eczema 70, 84
 see also named chemicals
chemist
 checking products with 133
 see also over the counter
 medications
cherries 136

chest deformities in children 51
chest symptoms 9
 see also coughing; tightness in
 chest; wheezing *etc.*
chickenpox 6, 86
childhood infections 6
children
 and allergy vaccine 11
 asthma treatments for 49–50
 beef 137
 bone strength 49
 chest deformities 51
 chickenpox virus 86
 common cold virus 32
 cot death 156–7
 cow's milk allergy 81–2, 126,
 127, 134, 138–9, 142–3
 dermatitis in 67
 diet and eczema 80–2, 138
 eczema in 66–7, 70–2, 81–2,
 85–6, 199–200, 138, 202
 efficacy of medication for
 asthma 49
 eggs allergy 127–8, 134, 137,
 145–6
 exclusion diet 237
 food allergies 126, 127–9, 139
 growth 38, 49, 51, 52, 53, 113
 immune system in 135
 inhalers for asthma 42–3,
 49–50, 51–3, 197–8, 204
 medication by mouth 42
 outgrowing allergies 135, 170
 peanut allergy 129, 141–2,
 143–4
 refused entry to nursery school
 198
 responsibility for own
 treatment 214–15
 and school examinations 202–3
 and tobacco smoke 220

children *(continued)*
    under-achievement in school
        51, 97
    see also babies; school
Children's Charter 198
Chinese cuisine 147, 164, 165
Chinese therapy 241
chlorine in swimming pools 73, 78
chlorofluorocarbons *see* CFCs
chocolate 136, 238
chromate 87
chromosomes 5, 10, 27, 249
chrysanthemums 87, 91, 181
cigarette smoke see tobacco
    smoke
cigarettes, formaldehyde in 87, 91
cimetidine 12
circulatory system, failure to
    work 152
city, living in the 103–4
Clarityn 108, 117
cleaning and animals 56–7, 234
clinics, specialist allergy 169
clothing 78
    and animal allergy 234–5
    crease-resistant 91
    and eczema 71, 200
    and pollen allergy 231
    trapping insects 169
cloxacillin 171
co-factors (environmental) 20, 249
co-ordination in using inhalers 42,
    44, 45, 49
cobalt 37, 87
cocoa 136
coeliac disease 122, 134, 148–50,
    213, 238, 249, 269
Coeliac Society, The 150
coffee 37
coins 91
cola 136

cold air 20, 32, 62
cold sore virus and eczema 86
colds and allergies 20, 28
    general anaesthetics 205–6
colic 13
collapse through anaphylaxis 130,
    131, 152
colophony 176
common cold 32, 95–6, 101
Community Health Council 125
compensation, industrial 37, 173
complementary therapies 114,
    239–46, 249
computer work 182–3
concentration impairment 97
condoms, latex 209
confiscation of medication when
    travelling abroad 192
conjunctivitis 97, 102, 249
    occupational 174
constipation 52
contact dermatitis see dermatitis
contact lenses
    and pollen allergy 231
    problems 102
contraceptives 209
    the pill and hayfever treatment
        113
cookbooks for people with
    allergies 213
cooking affecting food allergies
    135
corn 134, 136, 237
corticosteroids 40, 53, 76, 112,
    239, 244
    see also steroids
cosmetics 87, 89, 90–1
    fragrance attracting insects 169
cot death (sudden infant death
    syndrome or SIDS) 156–7
cotton clothing 78

coughing 13
  activated by dry powder inhaler
    46–7, 48
  in asthma 30, 32, 38–9
  in food allergies 130
  from catarrh 101
  and tobacco smoke 33–4
country, living in the 103
courgettes 134
crabs 136
cranial osteopathy 244–5
crayfish 136
creams, skin 200
creams versus ointments 74
crème fraîche 238
cromoglycate *see* sodium
  cromoglycate
Crosby capsule 270
crying 32
Cuprofen 33, 62, 64
cure for allergies 11
curtains 222, 224
custard 238
Customs and Excise, confiscation
  of medication 192
Cutivate 75
cyanosis *see* blueness
cypress, Leyland 181

dairy products 123, 124
  see also milk, cow's
daisy family and allergies 91, 232
dander
  cat 17, 56, 94, 233, 249
  dog 17, 94, 249
danger
  of anaphylaxis 152
  of asthma 51
daphne shrub 181
death
  from anaphylaxis 156, 169

death *(continued)*
  from asthma 51
  from food allergies 129
decongestant nasal sprays 107,
  110–11, 112–13, 249
decongestant tablets 107, 111,
  116, 249
deep sea diving 36
dehumidifiers 59
Department of Health
  investigation 10
  occupational triggers
    information 37
  publications 191, 277, 278
depigmentation of skin 83–4, 250
depilatory creams 133
depression 9
dermatitis 9, 23, 62, 65, 87–92, 250
  allergens causing 87
  in catering work 183–4
  difference between dermatitis
    and eczema 66–7
  occupational 174
  treatment 67
  see also names of individual
    substances
Dermatophagoides
  pteronyssimus (house dust
  mite) 18, 221, *221*
desensitization 11, 54, 114, 250
  enzyme potentiated (EPD) 246
  injections 114, 169–70
desserts 238
detergents 70, 207
devices
  for treatment of asthma 42–8
  see also individual names
dextrose 124
diagnosis, importance of correct 8
  see also tests
diarrhoea 8, 13, 16, 101, 132

diarrhoea *(continued)*
  caused by cow's milk 123
  and coeliac disease 148–9
diary
  of asthma symptoms 40
  of particular foods eaten 131,
    139
diet
  balanced 124, 144
  and development of allergic
    problems 220
  diary of 131, 139
  and eczema 70, 80–3
  egg-free 238
  elimination/exclusion 140, 144,
    236, 237
  help with cost of special 213
  in hospital 207
  milk-free 237–8
  strictness with 16
  wheat-free 238
digestion problems 11, 13, 122–3
diphtheria vaccines 153
discrimination at work on health
  grounds 178
Diskhaler 46–7, 47
diurnal variation in peak flow
  measurement 41, 250
DIY hobbies as trigger for asthma
  34
dizziness 130, 131, 155
doctor
  abroad 189
  anaphylaxis treatment 131
  diagnosing asthma 37–8, 39
  diagnosing atopy 5
  examination for allergy 15, 16,
    37–8, 106
  hospital treatment by 12
  interpretation of tests 142
  and self-management plans 51

doctor *(continued)*
  skin prick testing 71, 81
  and symptoms of allergy 14–15
  urgent need to visit 42, 184
dogs 13, 17, 78, 234
dosage
  frequency 12, 50–1
  gradual increase in
    desensitization 12
  maintenance level 12
  minute 11
  of preventer medications 52
  see also individual medications
dried food 58
dried milk solids 238
driving safely
  after adrenaline treatment 161
  and hayfever 108, 115–16
  see also car
drowsiness when taking certain
  medications 55, 108, 118
drugs 18
  adrenaline 145
  allergy to drugs 11
  anaesthetic 208
  antibiotics 63–4
  antihistamines 7, 49
  antivirus 86
  by inhalers 42–3
  corticosteroids 49
  dangerous combination 112–13
  hayfever 106–8
  injected 63
  limited availability abroad
    191–2
  as non-allergic causes of
    urticaria 62
  powder form 46–7
  reaction 7
  suitability for inhaler devices
    45–7

drugs *(continued)*
  as triggers in asthma 33
  two names for each 192
dry mouth 52
dry powder inhaler device *see*
  Diskhaler; Turbohaler
dryness of skin 66, 69, 72
duodenal ulcers 12
duration of treatment 11–12, 13
dust 36, 37, 221
  see also house dust mites;
    housing conditions
duvets 78, 224
dyestuffs 63, 87, 179

E45 cream 182
E number 102 food additive 58,
  63, 138
ear, nose and throat specialist
  118
earrings 90–1
ears
  blockage owing to allergy 118
  eczema behind ears 66
  pierced 90–1
eating out *see* restaurant food
eczema 4, 9, 23, 62, 250
  and animals 186–7
  causes 69–72
  degrees of severity 69
  diet 80–3
  difference between eczema and
    dermatitis 66–7
  duration 62
  and family toiletries 209
  and food allergies 130, 138–9
  on hands only 67
  herbal medicines 243–4
  homeopathy 246
  in hospital 207
  and house dust mites 19

eczema *(continued)*
  and hyper-IgE syndrome 12
  hypnosis 246
  incidence *21*
  infantile 20–1, 66, 68–9
    `growing out of it' 66, 68
  living with eczema 83–7
  not contagious 65
  parts affected in mild cases 66
  prevention 69–70
  related to asthma and hayfever
    68, 72, 202
  skin protection treatment 200
  and swimming 199–200
  treatment 67, 72–80
  triggers 78–9
  worsening in children 70–1, 77,
    202
effectiveness of inhalers reduced
  by use 48
eggs 27, 59, 69, 80, 81, 82
  allergy in children 127–8, 134,
    137, 138, 145–6
  cause of problems 162, 236
  egg-free diet 238
  raw 135
elbows, eczema of 66
elderly people 10, 28
  dermatitis in 67
elimination/exclusion diet 140,
  144, 236, 237, 250–1
Elocon 75
emergency treatment
  abroad 191
  acute food allergy/anaphylaxis
    130–1, 152–3, 157–61, 165
  bee and wasp stings 162
  nosebleeding 100
  and schools 198–9, 201
emollients 67, 72, 73, 200, 202,
  250

emotional factors 19, 32, 183, 210
employers' responsibility and
    allergies 174
emulsifying ointment 73
environmental factors 19–20, 27,
    218–19
    and asthma 29, 53–4, 68
    testing 270
enzyme
    as additive 78
    for digestion 122
enzyme detergents 178
EPD (enzyme potentiated
    desensitization) 246
epinephrine (adrenaline) 159, 247,
    251
Epipen injection device 159, *159*,
    165, 168–9
epoxy resins 37
Erymax 113
Erythromid 113
erythromycin 113
Erythroped 113
essential oils in aromatherapy 242
Euphrasia officinalis (eyebright)
    114
European Union
    CFCs regulations 108
    food regulations 133
Eustachian tubes (ear and nose)
    118
evening primrose oil for eczema
    79
excitement 32
excluding problem foods 82–3,
    236
exclusion/elimination diet 140,
    145
exercise 20
    exercise-induced anaphylaxis
    166

exercise *(continued)*
    and pollen allergy 230
    and tightness in chest 96
    as trigger for asthma 32, 194
    see also sport
exposure to allergens 20, 27
    reducing 106
external factors and asthma 55
eyebright homeopathic remedy
    for hayfever 114
eyes 9, 13, 63
    anti-allergy drops 107, 110–11,
    111, 116
    bathing 102, 110
    blurred vision 52
    computer work 182
    contact lenses 102
    dark appearance below eyes 97
    pain beneath eyes 99
    red and swollen 101–2, 179
    solutions for bathing 107, 110,
    111
    watery 95, 97, 101–2, 179

fabric softeners 87, 91
face
    itching and redness 182
    steroid cream on 75
    swelling of 80
factory work 175–6
fainting, through food allergy 131,
    155
families
    allergies running in 5, 14, 26,
    28, 68, 131
    quality of life for 51
    see also atopy; inheritance
fast food chains 166
fatigue 9
fats 238
fear of injections 16, 159, 171, 241

feathers 224
fevers 20
fields 60
finance and allergies 212–13
Fire Service 36
first aid
  acute food allergy 130–1
  anaphylaxis 130–1, 152–3, 165
  bee and wasp stings 162
  nosebleeding 100
fish (white) 62, 80, 134
  for babies 126
  cause of problems 162, 164, 236
  see also shellfish
flooring and dust 60
flour 37, 149–50
flowers 85
  see also Bach flower remedies;
    herbal medicines; pollen
    calendar; trees
Floxapen 171
flucloxacillin 171
fluticasone propionate 75
flying 189, 193
food
  additives 58, 235
    see also individual brand
    names
  avoidance 236
  colourings 63, 124, 138
  convenience and pre-prepared
    83, 124, 133, 145–6
  families 136
  intolerance 121, 122–3
  kinds rarely responsible for
    allergies 134
  labelling 133, 138
  losing enjoyment of 118
  main problem foods 236–7
  poisoning 123, 184
  preparation 135

food (continued)
  processed 29, 133
  reaction to 7, 11, 33, 57, 121–2
  school meals 201
  sensitivity rather than true
    allergy 121, 123
food allergies 23, 57–8, 80,
  120–50, 235–8
  challenge tests see challenge
    tests
  closely related foods 136
  cure 132–3
  diagnosis 137–42
  diary of diet 83, 139, 251
  difficulty of diagnosis 81, 82–3,
    131, 139–40
  and eczema 138
  exclusion diet 82–3, 139, 140
  explanation 121–9
  on holiday abroad 85
  inherited 126–7
  living with 142–8
  multiple severe 145
  only one or two 125–8
  precise use of the term 122
  predisposing factors 126
  reintroducing excluded foods
    82–3
  severity of 134
  symptoms 130–2
  time between eating and
    symptoms 131–2
  triggers for 132–7
  true 120–1
  see also individual foods
foot massage 243
forearms, dermatitis of 65
foreign holidays see holidays;
  travel
forestry work 181
formaldehyde 67, 87, 91

fragrances
    attracting insects 169
    and dermatitis 87, 89, 91
    and eczema 70, 78
free prescriptions 212
French beans 136
frequency of symptoms 14, 39–40
fried rice 238
fromage frais 238
fructose 124
fruit 124, 134, 136, 237
    for babies 126
fumes, exposure to 9, 33, 36, 39
fungi 181
fur 56, 60, 70, 78
furnishings, soft 18
furniture, upholstered 226

garage work and dermatitis 185–6
gardening
    and dermatitis 91–2, 180–1
    and hay fever 117, 231–2
    precautions against bees and
        wasps 168
garlic remedy for hayfever 114
gas boilers 60
gastrointestinal tract (gut) 130
gastroscope 269
GCSE examinations and stress
    202–3
gender, and allergies 12, 29, 67,
    129
general health 35
generic names for drugs 192, 251
genes 5, 20, 27, 251
geographical areas and allergies
    218–19
giving yourself an injection 161
glazing on baked foods 238
gloves
    gardening 92

gloves *(continued)*
    protective 179, 184, 185
    rubber 67, 87, 92
glue ear 118
gluten 126, 134, 149, 251
gluten-free foods 149–50, 213
Government Acts relating to
    working conditions 172
GP (general practitioner) *see*
    doctor
grains 37, 238
grapefruit 136
grasses *see* pollen
gravy 238
gravy mixes 58
green beans 134, 136
groundnuts 166
    see also arachis; peanuts
growth, when taking inhaled
    steroids 53

H_1 blockers 12
H_2 blockers 12, 13
hair analysis test 270
hair or fur from dogs 17, 70
hairdressing chemicals 88, 184–5
hands
    dermatitis 87–8, 178–9, 183–4,
        185
    eczema only 67
    red and swollen 65
    trembling 52
Hay-Crom Hay Fever eye drops
    110
hayfever 4, 9, 57, 93–119, 251
    in adolescence 20
    all-year-round 94–5
    antibiotics not helpful 101
    and asthma 95
    complementary remedies 114
    control without drugs 105

hayfever *(continued)*
densensitization treatment 11
different from common cold 96
during pregnancy 117
and dyestuffs at work 179–80
early treatment essential 104
and eczema 66
and EPD treatment 246
explanation 94
and general anaesthetics 206
and homeopathy 245–6
incidence of *21*, 93
living in the country or city
103–4
living with 115–19
perennial 94–5
and school examinations 202–3
symptoms 97–102
treatment 97, 106–14, 107–8,
116–17
triggers 103–6
variable symptoms 104–5
see also pollens
Hayfever in the Garden 23
hazards in the workplace 174
hazelnut chocolate 136
headaches 99, 123
health, general 35
health costs, help with 212–13
health and employment 177–8
health questionnaires in job
applications 177–8
Health and Safety at Work Act
(1974) 174
Health and Safety Executive 37,
174, 175
hearing affected by allergy 118
heart
irregularities in beat 113
palpitations 130
rapid rate of 31

heart *(continued)*
and weight problem 54
heart rate and medication 52
heat 62, 84
heating of houses 18, 29, 60
herbal medicines 243–4
hereditary conditions *see*
inheritance
Hismanal 108, 117
histamines 7, 12, 95, 98, 251
see also antihistamines
hives 23, 62, 251
hoarseness 52
hobbies, and asthma 34
holidays 28, 39
and allergies 189–96, 231
and food allergies 130–1
and hayfever 115, 231
improving eczema 79–80, 85
precautions to consider 190–1
skin problems 84–5
homeopathy 114, 245–6
hooks and eyes 90
hormones 158
horses 35
hospital
abroad 191
anaphylaxis while in-patient
207
going into 205–8
latex allergy in 207
observation for severe allergic
reaction 161, 167
treatment in 12, 142, 152
hot dogs 238
hotel bedding and linen 85
house dust mites 13, 15, 17,
18–19, 221–8, *221*, 251
and altitude 219
and asthma 29, 34, 58, 60
and eczema 60, 70, 71, 78, 85–6

house dust mites *(continued)*
and hayfever 94, 105
and housework 221–3
in office buildings 183
household utensils 91
houses 18, 69
and asthma 59–60
and pollen allergy 231
housework and house dust mites
221–3
humidity 70, 84, 85, 226
and asthma 34, 35, 59
and house dust mites 222, 226
hyacinths 181
hydrocortisone 75
hydrolysed vegetable protein 166
hypnosis 246
hypoallergenic products 89–90,
91, 252

ibuprofen 33, 64
after bee or wasp stings 162
ice cream 135, 238
icepack after removing stings 162
identification for people with
allergies 154, 169, 213–14
identity cards 214
idiopathic anaphylaxis 165, 252
IgA 6, 149
IgD 6
IgE 4, 6, 10, 12, 14, 252
food allergy 121
IgG 5–6, 149
IgM 5
immune system 4, 252
how it works 5–7, 135
immunoglobulin, types A,D,E,G,M
see IgA; IgD; IgE; IgG; IgM
immunological disorders 122
immunotherapy 11–13, 54, 114,
169–70, 252

individual variation of symptoms
13
industrial waste products 33
infantile eczema *see* eczema,
infantile
infants
asthma treatments for 49–50
cot death 156–7
eczema in *see* infantile eczema
infection, natural protection
against 14
inflammation 65, 252
of airways in asthma 25, 43, 49,
57
of nose
in food allergies 132
in hayfever 94, 98
as result of allergy 10, 14, 15, 65
as root of all allergies 218
see also dermatitis; skin
information
asking for 167
asthma and schoolchildren 43
baby foods 126
food additives 138
from employer 174
giving it to others 167
occupational triggers 37
pharmaceutical companies 192
for schools about asthma 197
to employer on one's health 178
inhalation of allergens 13
inhalers
access essential for children
198
adrenaline 131, 145, 160
for asthma 7, 8
and breathlessness 31
co-ordination in use of 42, 44,
45, 49
correct use 43–8, 252

inhalers *(continued)*
 metered dose 43–6, *44*, 49, 160,
  253
 types of 42–8, 49
 use in hospital 206
 use in pregnancy 53
inhalers versus nasal sprays 108
inheritance 5, 19–22, 26, 28, 68–9
 and food allergies 127, 143
 and workplace allergies 173
 see also atopy
injections 11, 12
 adrenaline 131, 157–8, 160–1,
  165
 desensitizing 114
 fear of 159, 171, 241
 how to give 161, 167
 side effects 158–9
injury 5, 14
insect bites on holiday, avoidance
 of 196
insect stings 11
 reaction to 7
insects 37, 153, 168, 195
 see also bee stings; wasp stings
insulation in houses 69
insurance, medical (holiday) 190–1
Intal 52
intolerance as opposed to allergy
 7–8, 15, 252
intradermal testing 261
intrinsic factors and asthma 55
ionizers 59
ipatropium 49, 52
irritability 14, 15, 26
 in hayfever 97–8
irritable bowel syndrome 123
itching
 ears 98
 eyes, nose and throat 97, 98,
  101, 104

itching *(continued)*
 lips and tongue 130
 skin 6, 7, 14, 15, 63, 64, 65
  in eczema 72, 74, 80
  in food allergies 132
 ivy 87, 181

jean studs 87, 90–1
jewellery 87, 90–1
 for identification of allergy 169,
  214
job applications and health
 questionnaires 177–8
jobs and asthma *see* occupational
 triggers in asthma

Kenalog 113–14
ketotifen 12, 49, 68
knees, eczema behind 66

labelling of products 124, 133,
 138, 146–7, 166, 179
 and exclusion diet 237
lactase in digestion 8
lactose 8, 124, 238
ladybird bites 17
lamb 134
lancets used in skin prick testing
 16, 259
langoustines 136
language problems on holiday 189
lanolin
 and dermatitis 87
 and eczema 70, 77–8
latex allergy 67, 88, 178–9, 209,
 253
laughing 32
leather, tanned 87
legumes 134, 135, 136, 253
lemon meringue pie 147
lemons 136

length of treatment *see* duration of treatment
lethargy 97
leukocytotoxic tests 271
Leyland cypress 181
lifestyle, and asthma 20
lilies 181
lima beans 136
limes 136
lips, swelling of 130, 132, 139, 144, 159–60
liquid preparations 108
liquorice 136
living room, treatment for house dust mites 227
lobster 136
loganberries 136
loratadine 108, 117
loss of consciousness 154, 155
lumps, itchy 63
lungs 14
  affected by asthma 25–6, 57
  affected by dyestuffs 179–80
  becoming accustomed to inhalers 48
  function tests 38, 267–8
  and hayfever symptoms 57, 96
  inhalation of allergens 13
  and peak flow meter 40–2
  and tobacco smoke 33–4
  and weight problem 54

Magnapen 171
make-up *see* cosmetics
maltodextrin 124
mango 136
manipulation *see* osteopathy
margarine and low fat spreads 238
marrows 134
massage 242–3
matches 87

materials for clothing 78
mattresses 18, 70, 78, 86, 222, 223
mayonnaise 135, 238
measurement of air in lungs *see* peak flow meter
meat 134, 137
mecaptobenzothiazole 87, 92
Medic-Alert Foundation 214
medical care abroad 189–91
medical history 131, 178
medical treatment *see* doctor; drugs; hospital; treatment
medication
  always to hand on holiday 191
  availability abroad 191–2
  importance of regularity 29–30, 43
  liquid 50
  see also treatment
Medihaler-Epi 160
memory loss 9
menstrual periods, and asthma 29, 40
meringues 238
metals 37
metered dose inhalers *see* inhalers, metered dose
micro-organisms and immune system 5
migraine 123
milk
  condensed 238
  drinks 238
  evaporated 238
  soya-based 213
milk (cow's)
  allergy 135, 138, 142–3, 236
  allergy and beef 137
  for infants 126
  intolerance 8, 15–16, 16, 27, 122
  milk-free diets 237–8

milk (cow's) *(continued)*
  in pregnancy 143
  trigger for asthma 33, 58, 59,
    142–3
  trigger for eczema 69, 80–2,
    142–3
  trigger for urticaria 62
milk products 122–3, 237–8
millet 136
missing school 204
MMR (measles, mumps, rubella)
  vaccine 137
model building as trigger for
  asthma 34
mometasone furoate 75
monitoring asthma symptoms 38,
  39
moodiness 15
mould spores 104
moulds 34, 181
mouth
  medication by 42
  swelling of 80, 130, 154
moving house 59–60
moving house to help with allergy
  problems 218–19
mowing the lawn and pollen
  allergy 231, 232
mucus 6, 7, 13, 26
  in hayfever 98, 101
multiple chemical sensitivity 9
multiple RAST 264
multivitamin liquid containing
  peanut oil 133

narcissus 181
narrowing of airways 25–6
nasal decongestants 96
nasal polyps 96
nasal sprays 57, 107, 108
  and driving ability 116

nasal sprays *(continued)*
  steroid 112
  using 108, *109*, 110
National Asthma Campaign 43, 197
National Asthma and Respiratory
  Training Centre 43, 197
natural fibres 78
nausea 130, 132, 155
nebulisers, for treatment of
  asthma 50, *50*, 194, 253
nedocromil 253
needles
  fear of injections *see* injections
  in skin prick testing 16
nettle rash 23, 62, 134, 139, 253
neutralisation-provocation testing
  (Miller technique) 271
newsprint 87, 91
nickel 67, 87, 90–1
nitrogen oxides 104
non-protein allergens 18
nose 9, 13, 14, 57, 63
  bleeding 99–100
  blockage 99, 100, 118
  hayfever symptoms 94–6, 98
  inflammation 132
  nasal polyps 96
  runny 95–6, 97, 98, 118–19,
    179
  see also rhinitis
nosebleeding in hayfever 99–100
Nurofen 33, 62, 64
nursery school, children refused
  entry 198
nurses, and diagnosis of asthma
  37–8
nuts 58, 59, 62, 80, 134, 135
  common cause of anaphylactic
    reactions 162
  see also peanuts
oats 134, 150

observation for severe reaction to treatment 12
obstruction of upper airway 152
occupational allergies 72–87, 253
  how they happen 174
  whom to consult 175
occupational triggers 33, 36–7, 39, 88
occurrence of symptoms 13–14
office work 182–3
oil seed rape 104
ointments
  emulsifying 73
  versus creams 74
onion remedy for hayfever 114
operating machinery while drowsy 108
Opticrom Allergy eye drops 110
Optrex 110
oral challenge tests 266
oral thrush 52
oranges 136
osteopathy 244–5
osteoporosis 52, 113
over the counter medications (OTC) 75, 107, 108, 113, 171, 212–13, 253
overweight problem and asthma 54
oxitropium 52
Oxivent 52
ozone 104

packet foods 58
painkillers 33, 63–4
paint fumes 39
painting and decorating 187
paints, reaction to 187
paleness of skin on face and knees 83–4
palpitations 130

pancakes 238
parabens 77–8, 87
paracetamol 62, 74, 100
  after bee or wasp stings 162
parachuting 194
parasites 5
passive smoking 33, 253
  see also tobacco smoke
pasta and noodles 238
patch testing 67, 88, 181, 253, 261–3, 262
Patient's Charter 125
pattern of asthma symptoms 40
peaches 136
peak expiratory flow 40, 176, 253, 267
peak flow measurement 31, 38, 40–2, 51
  dropping 42
  increasing variations 42
peak flow meter 38, 39, 40, 40, 176, 181, 253
  how to use 40–2
peanut oil 17, 133
peanuts 58, 126–7, 128, 129, 133, 134, 146–7
  adrenaline injection for 160–1
  allergy in early life 141–2, 143–4
  anaphylactic reactions from 153, 154, 163, 166, 208–9
  avoiding when on holiday 194–5
peas 136
Penbritin 171
penicillin 18, 62, 64
  anaphylactic reactions from 153, 170–1
  cause of anaphylactic reactions 162
peptic ulcers 12
perennial allergic rhinitis see rhinitis

perfume *see* fragrances
pet allergens *see* animals
petroleum jelly 118–19
pets *see* animals
pharmacy *see* chemist
phlegm *see* mucus
pillows 18, 78, 222, 224
pinto beans 136
Piriton 117
pistachio nuts 136
plants 85, 87, 91–2, 181
    aromatherapy 242–3
    herbal medicines 243
    see also gardening; pollens
plastics 9
platinum salts 178
playgroups, children refused
    entry 198
plums 136
poisoning, food 123
Police Service 36
pollen
    calendar 228–30, *229*, 254
    tests for allergy 104, 253–4
pollen count 34, 103, 104–5, 110,
    115, 254
    geographical distribution
        218–19
    staying indoors 230, 231
pollens 228–32, *229*
    commonsense measures to
        avoid 230–1
    description 103, 228
    and eczema 70
    grass 10, 13, 15, 20, 55, 60, 104
        variable symptoms 104–5
    and hayfever 94–5, 98, 101–2,
        104
    integral pollen filter in car 116
    oil seed rape 104
    plant 23, 34, 55, *229*

pollens *(continued)*
    tree 104, *229*
    weed 104
polymorphic light eruption 84
polyurethane 37
potatoes 134
potholing 194
powder
    desensitizing (nasal) 114
    milk 238
power supply abroad for
    nebuliser 194
predisposition to allergies *see*
    atopy; inheritance
prednisolone 49, 52, 76
pregnancy
    asthma attack during labour
        211
    and asthma treatment 53, 210
    and asthma worsening 210
    and food allergies 126–7, 143
    hayfever medications during
        107
    and hayfever worsening 117
    and tobacco smoke 220
prepared food 83, 124, 133,
    145–6
prescription charges 212–13
preservatives
    food 63, 137–8
    formaldehyde 91
pressure as trigger 62
preventers for asthma 35, 43, 198,
    254
    and general anaesthetics 205
    side effects of 52–3
    when to use 48, 193
    see also relievers for asthma
prickly heat 84
primula obconica 87, 181
protective clothing 179, 180, 187

protein
  and cooking 135
  sources of 81, 82, 124, 137
protein in allergens 17, 70
proteins, animal 178
provocation tests *see* challenge
  tests
psoralen *see* PUVA
psychosomatic symptoms 124–5,
  254
puddings 238
Pulmicort 52
PUVA (psoralen plus ultra-violet
  A) 80, 254

quality control and eating out 166

rabbits 78
radiation from computer screens
  182
radiators 60
radioallergosorbant test *see* RAST
rain reducing pollen count 231–2
ranitidine 13
rash
  itchy red 84
  mouth and throat 52
  skin 62–3, 87, 101
    duration of 64
raspberries 136
RAST 81, 82, 83, 139, 142, 163,
  254, 263–4
  advantage of 164
redness, as symptom 6, 7, 14, 87
relatives *see* families; inheritance
relaxation, therapy to induce
  242–3
relievers for asthma 31, 35, 43, 253
  before sexual intercourse 210
  failure to work 48
  two main types 51–2

relievers for asthma *(continued)*
  when to use 48–9, 53
  see also preventers for asthma
research
  antihistamines and eczema in
    babies 68
  desensitization 169–70
  EPD (enzyme potentiated
    desensitization) 246
  evening primrose oil 79
  genetic 22, 27
  herbal medicines 244
  prevention of allergies 219–20
  sick building syndrome 183
  vaccine against allergy 11
resistance to disease *see* immune
  system
respirator for use when
  decorating 187
respiratory infections 18, 27, 32
restaurant food 8, 133, 147–8,
  166
rhinitis 4, 9, 11, 19, 23, 105, 247,
  254
  occupational 174
  vasomotor 96
rhinitis medicamentosa 96, 255
risks
  anaphylactic shock 155
  in asthma treatments 53
  with desensitization 11
  to other people from
    asthmatics 36
rosin 176
rubber products and dermatitis
  67, 87
runner beans 136
runny nose 95–6, 97, 98, 118–19,
  179
rye 134, 136, 150
Rynacron 107

safety at work 174, 175, 177, 179, 180
safety of steroid creams 74–6
salad cream 238
salbutamol 8, 38, 52
  for children 49
saliva 5
saliva from cats 17, 86, 106
salt water 73
sauces 238
  packet 58
sausages 238
scabs, dermatitis 87
scaling of skin 65–6
scampi 136
Scandinavian law on nickel 91
Schefflera 181
school 196–205
  asthma policy 204
  attitude to allergy treatments 198–9
  bullying affecting eczema 202
  children's responsibility for own treatment 214–15
  children's under-achievement in 51, 97
  danger of medication being locked away 196
  examination stress 202–3
  going to school with severe eczema 202
  immediate access to inhalers 198
  inhalers 42–3
  meals 201
  missing school through allergy 204
  special educational needs 204–5
  starting school with asthma 196–7

school (continued)
  stress at 79
  trips away from home 203
score card see diary
scratching of skin 65–6, 69
scuba diving and asthma 194
sea bathing 73
sea breezes and pollen count 115
seafood 58, 127
seasonal asthma 57
secretions, increased 6, 13, 15
self-catering holiday 194, 196
self-help goups 216
self-injection 161
self-management of asthma treatment 51, 255
sensitivity 8, 15
  multiple chemical 9
sensitizers, allergic 173, 255
sesame seeds 145
severity of allergy 7, 10, 28, 36–7
sex and pregnancy 208–12
  see also pregnancy
shakiness, in asthma treatment 8
shampoo 70, 78
shaving cream 209
sheets, plastic 225
shellfish 58, 62, 85, 126–7, 130, 134, 159–60
  anaphylactic shock from eating 153
  closely related foods 136
  common cause of problems 162, 164, 165–6, 236
  and exercise 166
shiatsu 242
shoes carrying cat allergen 57
shortness of breath see breathlessness
shrimps 136
sick building syndrome 183

side effects
  antibiotics 101, 255
  antihistamines 108
  asthma treatment 8, 51–3
  inhaled drugs 42
  nasal sprays 112
  steroid creams 74–6
sinuses
  infected 101, 255
  inflammation in 97
  pain in 99, 101
size of inhaler devices 45, 48
skin
  allergen entering through 14
  allergies 9, 61–92
  conditioning before swimming 200
  delicate or sensitive 84
  infections 65, 78, 79
  inflamed and broken 78, 86
  problems on holiday abroad 84–5
  and PUVA 80
  rash 62–3, 67–8, 101
  soreness around nose and mouth 118–19
  structure of 61–2
  thickening and scaling of 65
  see also dermatitis; itching
skin creams 60, 70, 72, 74, 77, 88
skin prick tests 15–16, 38, 55, 71, 141, 255–6
  for animal allergy 234
  description 259–61, 260
  dyestuffs allergy 180
  fear of 140–1
  food allergies 81, 82, 137, 139–40, 163
  for food allergies, advantage of 164
  intradermal 261

skin-prick tests (continued)
  in supermarkets 142
sleep 15, 51, 97, 99
sleepiness when taking certain medications 108
smell, loss of sense of 97, 118
smoking see tobacco smoke
sneezing 95, 97
soap 70, 72–3, 74, 78
  and dermatitis 87
  and eczema 209
sodium cromoglycate 52, 110, 145, 249
  nasal sprays 107
sodium metabisulphate 58
soft drinks 58
soft furnishings 18, 70
soldering flux 37, 176
solvents and allergies 179, 180, 185
sore throat in hayfever 99, 100
soreness, as symptom 14, 15
soup 58, 238
soya beans 134, 148
spacer devices for asthma treatment 45, 49, 52
spasm
  of airways muscles 26
  of bowel 13
special educational needs 204–5
specialist, referral to 125, 139, 144–5, 155, 164–5, 180, 184
spectacles
  frames 91
  and pollen allergy 231
spores 34, 181
sport, and asthma 29, 34–5
spray paints 37
sprays, for house dust mites 227
squash family 134
squid 136

staff associations 175
Staphylococcus, causing skin
   infection 79
starch 150
starch powder in rubber gloves
   92
state schools and medical needs
   of children 190
statistics 3
   age 10
   allergies at work 174
   anaphylactic shock 156
   asthma 24–5, 28–9
   conjunctivitis 102
   dermatitis 67
   diet and eczema 80
   eczema 61
   food allergens 235
   food allergies 121–2, 128–9
   gender and asthma 29
   hayfever *21*, 93, 95
   herbal medicines 243
   house dust mites 221
   latex allergy 92
   peanuts and anaphylactic
      shock 129
   pet allergens 233
   scale of the problem 22–3
   stings causing anaphylactic
      reactions 162
steroids
   anabolic 49, 53, 76, 112
   creams and emollients 67, 72,
      74, 77
      depigmentation effect 84
      safety of 74–6
   inhaled 7, 52–3
   Kenalog 113–14
   nasal sprays 112, 114
   oral 52
   tablet form 52, 160

sticking plasters 91
stomach cramp *see* abdominal
   discomfort or pain
stomach ulcers 12
stomach upsets 101
strawberries 136
stress
   and allergies 19, 70, 123
   and asthma 28, 175–6
   at school 79
   Bach flower remedies for 244
   and eczema 70, 78, 85, 202, 207
   when going into hospital 207–8
strimmers 92
stroking animals 86, 186
sucrose 124
sudden infant death syndrome
   (SIDS) 156–7
sugar 124
   see also lactose
suitability of inhalation devices 42
sulphites 63
sulphur dioxide 104
sunblock cream 85
sunglasses 110, 232
sunlight 62, 85
   effect on skin 84
   over-exposure to 80
support groups 216
*Supporting pupils with medical
   needs in schools* 204
swallowing, difficulty in 132
sweat and sweat glands 84
swelling
   airways 25–6, 152
   from bee and wasp stings 162
   lips and lining of mouth 130,
      132, 139, 144
   mouth and face 80, 130
   nose tissues 99
swimming 73

swimming *(continued)*
  care of skin before and after
    200–1
  and eczema 199–200
symptoms 13–19
  anaphylaxis 153–4
  of bad asthma attack 31
  details of 14–15
  diary of 40, 139, 168–9, 256
  food allergies 130–2
  hayfever 97–102
  how they occur 13–14
  improvement in 15
  irregularity of asthma 29–30
  monitoring 38, 39
  prevention in asthma 43
  variation in asthma 30
Syntaris Hayfever nasal spray 107
synthetics 9
syringe for adrenaline injection
  159, *159*

tablets
  prednisolone 52
  for severe reaction 158
tangerines 136
Tartrazine 58, 63
taste, sense of 118
tayberries 136
teachers
  asthma policy 204
  coping with pupils' asthma
    196–8
  pupils' use of inhalers 42–3,
    197–8
  school meals 201
  see also school
teas, herbal 244
tendency to develop allergic
  disorders 4, 12, 26
tenderness, as symptom 6

terbutaline 52
terfenadine 108, 112–13
tests
  applied kinesiology 270
  for asthma 38
  auricular cardiac reflex 270
  blood 263–5
  choosing most suitable ones
    258–9
  environmental 270
  food challenge 122, 131, 140,
    163–4, 266–7
  hair analysis 270
  intradermal 261
  leukocytotoxic 271
  lung function 267–8
  neutralisation-provocation
    (Miller technique) 271
  patch *260*, 261–3
  peak expiratory flow 267–8
  RAST 263–4
  reasons for testing 257–8
  skin prick 15–16, 259–61
  for true food allergies 123, 124,
    163
  Vega 271
  see also individual type names
tetanus vaccines 153
textiles, working with 179–80
Thai cuisine 147
therapist, complementary 240
thickening of skin 65
thinning of bones *see*
  osteoporosis
thiurams 87, 92
throat, allergic reaction in 63
thrush, oral 52
tightness in chest 33, 39–40, 96,
  179, 187
timing of symptoms 14
Timentin 171

tingling of lips and tongue 130, 165–6
tiredness 15, 97
tissue damage in allergy 14
tobacco smoke 18, 20, 27, 33, 220
  and asthma 29, 33–4, 193
toiletries *see* fragrances; soaps
tolerance of body to allergen 11
tongue, swelling of 132, 159–60
total allergy syndrome 9–10
toys, soft 18, 70–1, 222, 225
trade unions 175
traffic fumes 33, 59
travel, and allergies 189–96
Traveller's Guide to Health 191
treatment
  asthma 42–54
  careful choice of 10–11
  changes in 41
  changing your own dosage 50–1
  dermatitis 67
  duration of 11–12, 13
  eczema 67
  folly of stopping 192–3
  hayfever 106–14
  lack of 10, 14
  peak flow meter in assessment
    of 41, 181
  preventers and relievers for
    asthma 43
  regularity 28
  sudden stopping 52, 53
  to interrupt allergy process 7
  to suppress effects of histamine
    7
tree pollen 60, *229*, 232
trembling of muscles 52
triggers
  allergens 16–19, 62–3
  asthma 26, 32–7, 49, 54, 55
  eczema 78–9

triggers *(continued)*
  food allergies 132–7
  hayfever 103–6
Triludan 108, 112
trimethoprim, reaction to 64
trivialisation of allergies 215
tulips 181
Turbohaler 47–8, *47*
turkey 134
twins and food allergies 127

ultra-violet light 80
unconsciousness 154
unperfumed products 89
upholstery 226
upper respiratory tract infections
  32
urinary infection 63
urine, difficulty in passing 52
urticaria 9, 23, 57, 62–3, 134, 256
  allergic causes 62–3
  difference between urticaria
    and skin allergies 62–3
  in food allergies 130
  non-allergic causes 62–3
  and sunlight 84

vaccine
  against allergy 11
  MMR 137
vaccines, anaphylactic reactions
  from 153
vacuum cleaning 222–4, 225, 233,
  234
  see also cleaning
variation in peak flow
  measurement 41
Vaseline 118–19
Vega testing 271
vegetable dusts (coffee, grains
  and flour) 37

vegetable oils, labelling of 133, 166
vegetables 134
vegetarianism and cosmetic testing 89–90
ventilation 226–7
  buildings 18, 60, 183
  cars 116
  in rooms being decorated 187
Ventolin 8, 38, 49, 52
veterinary work 186
virus infections 5, 63, 70
Vividrin 107
  eye drops 110
Volumatic inhaler 45, 45
vomiting 13, 123, 130, 132, 142

walnuts 136
warning signs of bad asthma attack 31
washing of bedding and soft furnishings 224, 231
washing powders 69, 70, 78, 85
wasp stings 11, 62, 155, 162
  avoiding being stung 168–9, 170
  desensitization 169–70
  emergency treatment for anaphylactic reaction 157–8
water as trigger 62
watery motions see diarrhoea
watery secretions 6, 13
weaning and food allergies 126
weather
  and asthma 34, 57
  and eczema 71, 84–5
  and pollen count 104–5, 115, 130
weed pollens see pollens, weed
'weeping' of skin 66
weight and asthma 54
wheat 80, 124, 134, 150, 237

wheat (continued)
  food for babies 126
wheezing 13, 80, 256
  in anaphylaxis 152
  in asthma 20, 32, 201–2
  during sexual intercourse 209–10
  in food allergies 130, 132
whey 238
white blood cells 6
windpipe (trachea) 96, 101
wine 58, 123
wood dusts 37
woollen clothing 78
work
  allergies at see occupational allergies
  environment see occupational triggers in asthma
  factory 175–6
worms (parasitic) 6
wrists, eczema of 66

yoghurt 126, 238

Zaditen 49
zinc 91
zip fasteners 87, 90
Zirtek 108, 118
Zovirax 86

Have you found **Allergies at your fingertips** practical and useful? If so, you may be interested in other books from Class Publishing.

Asthma at your fingertips
NEW SECOND EDITION £11.95
Dr Mark Levy, Professor Sean Hilton and Greta Barnes MBE

This book shows you how to keep your asthma – or your family's asthma – under control, making it easier to live a full, happy and healthy life.

'This book gives you the knowledge. Don't limit yourself.'
Adrian Moorhouse MBE, Olympic Gold Medallist

High blood pressure at your fingertips £11.95
Dr Julian Tudor Hart

The author uses all his 26 years of experience as a general practitioner and blood pressure expert to answer your questions on high blood pressure.

'Readable and comprehensive information.'
Dr Sylvia McLaughlan, Director General, The Stroke Association

Diabetes at your fingertips
THIRD EDITION £11.95
Professor Peter Sönksen, Dr Charles Fox and Sister Sue Judd

461 questions on diabetes are answered clearly and accurately – the ideal reference book for everyone with diabetes.

'I will certainly recommend it to my patients . . . I think it is brilliant.'
Robert Tattersall, Professor of Clinical Diabetes, Queen's Medical Centre, Nottingham

Parkinson's at your fingertips
£11.95
Dr Marie Oxtoby and Professor Adrian Williams

Full of practical help and advice for people with Parkinson's disease and their families.

'A super DIY manual for patients and carers.'
Dr Bernard Dean

Heart health at your fingertips
NEW! £11.95
Dr Graham Jackson

Everything you need to know to keep your heart healthy – and live life to the full! This practical handbook, written by a leading cardiologist, answers all your questions about heart conditions – from diagnosis to treatment and from work to relationships.

Cancer information at your fingertips
NEW SECOND EDITION £11.95
Val Speechley and Maxine Rosenfield

Recommended by the Cancer Research Campaign, this book provides straightforward, practical and positive answers to all your questions about cancer.

Alzheimer's at your fingertips
NEW! £11.95
Harry Cayton, Dr Nori Graham and Dr James Warner

At last – a book that tells you everything you need to know about Alzheimer's and other dementias.

'An invaluable contribution to understanding all forms of dementia.'
Dr Jonathan Miller CBE, President of the Alzheimer's Disease Society

Your child's epilepsy: a parent's guide £9.95
Dr Richard Appleton, Brian Chappell and Sister Margaret Beirne

If your child has epilepsy you will find this practical handbook indispensable.

'Of enormous value to any parent.'
Professor David Chadwick, The Walton Centre for Neurology and Neurosurgery

PRIORITY ORDER FORM

Cut out or photocopy this form and send it (post free in the UK) to:

Class Publishing Priority Service
FREEPOST (no stamp needed)
London W6 7BR

Tel: 01752 202301

Fax: 01752 202333

Please send me urgently
(tick boxes below)

Post included
price per copy
(UK only)

☐ **Allergies at your fingertips** £14.95
(ISBN 1 872362 52 4)

☐ **Asthma at your fingertips** £14.95
(ISBN 1 872362 67 2)

☐ **High blood pressure at your fingertips** £14.95
(ISBN 1 872362 48 6)

☐ **Diabetes at your fingertips** £14.95
(ISBN 1 872362 49 4)

☐ **Parkinson's at your fingertips** £14.95
(ISBN 1 872362 47 8)

☐ **Heart health at your fingertips** £14.95
(ISBN 1 872362 77 X)

☐ **Cancer information at your fingertips** £14.95
(ISBN 1 872362 56 7)

☐ **Alzheimer's at your fingertips** £14.95
(ISBN 1 872362 71 0)

☐ **Your child's epilepsy: a parent's guide** £12.95
(ISBN 1 872362 61 3)

TOTAL: _____

Easy ways to pay
Cheque: I enclose a cheque payable to Class Publishing for £_____
Credit card: please debit my ☐ Access ☐ Visa ☐ Amex ☐ Switch
Number: _____ Expiry date: _____
Name _____
My address for delivery is _____

_____
Town _____ County _____ Postcode _____
Telephone number (in case of query) _____
Credit card billing address if different from above _____

_____
Town _____ County _____ Postcode _____

Class Publishing's guarantee: remember that if, for any reason, you are not satisfied with these books, we will refund
all your money, without any questions asked. Prices and VAT rates may be altered for reasons beyond our control.